EFT for BACK PAIN

D0807939

by Dawson Church

Emotional Freedom Techniques

www.EFTUniverse.com

Energy Psychology Press
3340 Fulton Rd, #442, Fulton, CA 95439
www.energypsychologypress.com

Cataloging-in-Publication Data

Church, Dawson, 1956–

EFT for back pain / by Dawson Church and 33 EFT practitioners, instructors, students, and users. — 2nd ed.

p. cm.

Includes index.

ISBN 978-1-60415-032-2

1. Backache—Alternative treatment. 1. Emotion-focused therapy. I. Title.

RD771.B217C73 2009

617.5'6406—dc22

Cover design by Victoria Valentine
Editing by Stephanie Marohn
Typesetting by Karin Kinsey
Typeset in Cochin and Adobe Garamond
Printed in USA by Bang Printing
Second Edition
10 9 8 7 6 5 4 3 2 1

Important note: While EFT (Emotional Freedom Techniques) has produced remarkable clinical results, it must still be considered to be in the experimental stage and thus practitioners and the public must take complete responsibility for their use of it. Further, Dawson Church is not a licensed health professional and offers the information in this book solely as a life coach. Readers are strongly cautioned and advised to consult with a physician, psychologist, psychiatrist, or other licensed health care professional before utilizing any of the information in this book. The information is based on information from sources believed to be accurate and reliable and every reasonable effort has been made to make the information as complete and accurate as possible, but such completeness and accuracy cannot be guaranteed and is not guaranteed.

The author, publisher, and contributors to this book, and their successors, assigns, licensees, employees, officers, directors, attorneys, agents, and other parties related to them (a) do not make any representations, warranties, or guarantees that any of the information will produce any particular medical, psychological, physical, or emotional result; (b) are not engaged in the rendering of medical, psychological or other advice or services; (c) do not provide diagnosis, care, treatment, or rehabilitation of any individual; and (d) do not necessarily share the views and opinions expressed in the information. The information has not undergone evaluation and testing by the United States Food and Drug Administration or similar agency of any other country and is not intended to diagnose, treat, prevent, mitigate, or cure any disease. Risks that might be determined by such testing are unknown. If the reader purchases any services or products as a result of the information, the reader or user acknowledges that the reader or user has done so with informed consent. The information is provided on an "as is" basis without any warranties of any kind, express or implied, whether warranties as to use, merchantability, fitness for a particular purpose, or otherwise.

The author, publisher, and contributors to this book, and their successors, assigns, licensees, employees, officers, directors, attorneys, agents, and other parties related to them (a) expressly disclaim any liability for and shall not be liable for any loss or damage including but not limited to use of the information; (b) shall not be liable for any direct or indirect compensatory, special, incidental, or consequential damages or costs of any kind or character; (c) shall not be responsible for any acts or omissions by any party including but not limited to any party mentioned or included in the information or otherwise; (d) do not endorse or support any material or information from any party mentioned or included in the information or otherwise; and (e) will not be liable for damages or costs resulting from any claim whatsoever. The within limitation of warranties may be limited by the laws of certain states and/or other jurisdictions and so some of the foregoing limitations may not apply to the reader who may have other rights that vary from state to state. If the reader or user does not agree with any of the terms of the foregoing, the reader or user should not use the information in this book or read it. A reader who continues reading this book will be deemed to have accepted the provisions of this disclaimer.

Please consult qualified health practitioners regarding your use of EFT.

Contents

Introduction

I'm so glad you've picked up this book and are open to trying Emotional Freedom Techniques (EFT) for back pain. That openness to change is the start of the healing journey, and I expect to welcome you to the ranks of the thousands of people who've discovered how to live pain-free after learning EFT.

EFT is a simple technique. You'll learn it in the Quick Start section at the end of this chapter, and you'll be trying it on yourself within the next 30 minutes. Many people find immediate relief and wonder how a technique so quick and simple can yield such profound results. While rapid healing might seem miraculous, there are actually very good scientific explanations for how and why it happens. We'll cover these briefly in the first chapter.

Throughout this book, it won't be just me talking to you. *EFT for Back Pain* includes numerous stories written by some of the millions of people who've used EFT. Many of them have used it successfully for back pain, and contributed their experiences to the international story archive at EFT Universe (www.EFTUniverse.com). The accounts are as different from one another as people are different, yet the commonality is that EFT reduced or removed the sufferer's pain. The archive also contains stories about problems as diverse as PTSD (posttraumatic stress disorder), depression, phobias, public speaking anxiety, and obesity. Enter virtually any problem into the search engine on the site and you'll find someone who has successfully used EFT to resolve that problem.

The Role of Stress in Healing

How is a single technique able to solve so many problems? The reason is that they all have one component in common, and that ingredient is stress. Stress makes every problem worse. Suppose you're trying unsuccessfully to lose weight. You certainly need an appropriate diet and exercise program, but you are also probably stressed. You've tried many diets in the past and all have failed. You feel stress about exercising, and about not exercising enough. You're stressed about your appearance, and about what other people think of you. Your body isn't as flexible or mobile as it would be at your ideal weight, which stresses you more. All those stresses get between you and successful weight loss.

We find that when people eliminate their stress by using EFT, everything else they're trying to accomplish for their health and well-being simply works better. Stress makes it difficult to figure out which component holds the key to success. Without the stress, the real problem comes

（）

into sharp focus. Dozens of scientific studies show that EFT dramatically reduces stress in all its forms, and this helps restore both mental and emotional health.

A Grass-Roots Movement

The simplicity and effectiveness of EFT have made it one of the fastest-growing self-help methods ever offered. An examination of Google searches in June of 2013 showed that over nine million people searched for terms such as "EFT therapy" in that month alone. Over two million then visited one of the five largest EFT websites. There's no advertising campaign behind those numbers, and no drug company pushing the method. It's freely available online, which has led to a worldwide grass-roots movement as word of EFT has spread via the millions of people who use it. The movement is expanding daily because EFT works quickly and well, as you'll discover when you apply it to your own pain in the next few minutes.

Tapping

EFT is often called "tapping" because one of its key components is tapping with your fingertips on acupuncture points on your body. Acupuncture has been proven effective for a variety of problems in many scientific studies (Vickers et al., 2012). Those problems include physical symptoms such as pain as well as psychological problems such as PTSD.

While acupressure points ("acupoints," for short) can be stimulated by putting needles into them, they can also be stimulated without needles. One example is the Japanese massage method called Shiatsu, which massages the points. In this chapter we'll show you how to stimulate a series of acupoints on your own body by tapping on them with your fingertips. Pressure on acupoints seems to have much the same effect as needling them (Cherkin et al., 2009).

Acupuncture theory teaches that energy flows throughout the body via pathways called meridians. Disease can be caused by a blockage or interruption of that flow, and acupuncture or acupressure can be used to remove those blockages. In the early 1960s, an American chiropractor named George Goodheart discovered that he could successfully treat physical problems by tapping on acupoints (Adams & Davidson, 2011), and a clinical psychologist named Roger Callahan developed a system of acupoint tapping for psychological problems (Callahan, 2000). One of Callahan's students, Gary Craig, abbreviated Callahan's system and named it EFT (Craig & Fowlie, 1995).

My Own Back Pain Story

As the author of this book, I'm not just an EFT expert or an interested observer. I've suffered from back pain much of my life, and I'm amazed how effective EFT and exercise have been for me. One of my legs is 2 inches shorter than the other. This tilts my pelvis, just like the tilt of a stool with one leg 2 inches shorter than the others. To adjust, my lower back curves sharply, a common condition called scoliosis. Most people with severe scoliosis experience back pain.

I had periods of prolonged back pain in my 20s and in my 30s, with occasional bouts when it was so severe that I could not walk. During the bad periods, even trying to move brought an involuntary scream of pain from my mouth. An orthopedic surgeon recommended a built-up heel to adjust for at least some of the leg length difference, though he and several different chiropractors said there was a limited amount they could do for me and I was likely to be in pain all my life. Back pain became like background music for me—sometimes loud, sometimes soft, but always there.

One chiropractor explained to me how my stomach muscles helped support the back, so I bought a simple handheld ab wheel and began to use it daily. As my stomach muscles strengthened, my back pain lessened, and when I got serious about an exercise program and began going to the gym regularly, it lessened further.

A year or two after I learned EFT, I had a long and severe episode of back pain that lasted about 2 weeks. I tried the usual remedies, but they didn't work. So I looked for emotional contributors, as in this book I'll teach you to do. I discovered that I felt unsupported by members of my team at work, and identified some childhood events with a similar emotional flavor. "Unsupported"...back pain...get the connection? Your back is what supports your upper body, and I noticed the connection between my pain and my emotions around feeling unsupported.

I tapped on those events, and within minutes the pain was gone.

I can't claim that back pain has become a non-issue for me. I still can't walk long distances without my back aching, and I prefer upper-body workout routines. I have to lift and carry heavy items very carefully, and be mindful when I sit up, bend over, twist, or exercise at the gym—all so I don't put undue strain on my back. But for several years I've been virtually pain free. I stopped wearing the built-up shoe because it threw me off balance, and my back pain didn't return. Despite this seeming to be a "purely physical" condition, it turned out that emotions played a big part in my healing journey. Today I tap whenever I have any kind of pain. EFT is the method I turn to first, and it's usually effective.

Clinical EFT

EFT for Back Pain and the other books in this series are companions to *The EFT Manual* (Church, 2013). You'll find EFT's fundamental method, called the Basic Recipe, described in Chapter 2 of this book. That's the exact same form of EFT described in *The EFT Manual.* That form of EFT has been used in all those studies, and since it's been validated by much research, we call it Clinical EFT. There are many variants of EFT in the marketplace, but the only one that is backed by many years of scientific study is Clinical EFT. That's why if you do EFT as described in this book and *The EFT Manual,* you'll have the confidence of knowing you're using the exact same method that's been proven to work in that whole large body of research.

The books in this series also abide by the standards of the American Psychological Association (APA) in terms of style, ethics, and proof. The Clinical Psychology division of the APA (Division 12) published standards for "empirically validated treatments" (Chambless & Hollon, 1998), and Clinical EFT meets those standards for a wide variety of psychological problems including anxiety, depression, PTSD, and phobias (Feinstein, 2012).

Other Types of Pain

While this book focuses on back pain, EFT works for all types of pain: migraine headaches, bone fractures, premenstrual syndrome and menstrual cramps, muscle sprains, eyestrain, sports injuries, toothaches, indigestion, stings, cuts, burns, and bruises. All of these contain an element of stress, sometimes a large element. Once that has been tapped away, your perception of pain may be much less, or the pain may be gone altogether. The website TraumaTap.com offers a whole collection of stories by people who have used EFT for first aid, and their reports show than many types of emergency pain disappear rapidly after applying EFT. So if you have a form of pain other than back pain, you'll still find lots of useful ideas in this book.

In a study I did with 216 health care workers, we looked at their levels of pain after a 20-minute EFT session. On average, their pain went down by an astonishing 68% (Church & Brooks, 2010). The statistical significance of this result was so great that there was only one possibility in a thousand that the results could have been due to chance (p < .001). The study didn't discriminate between types of pain, just levels of pain. Across the whole spectrum of pain, the health care workers showed a two-thirds drop in their intensity levels. That's because there's a large emotional component in pain, no matter what the source.

Let's hear from some of the thousands of people who've used EFT for pain and other problems. You'll see that it can offer you dramatic results, and that it can work even when other methods have failed. In the first account, EFT Master and trainer Sophia Cayer tells the inspiring story of "Harry," who used EFT to resolve a back injury that had resulted in 42 years of back pain and 24 years on disability. Harry's case provides another example of how EFT can help what may seem to be a "purely physical" problem.

A New Life after 42 Years of Back Pain

By Sophia Cayer, EFT Master

You asked for a persistent tapper and "by Jove, I think we've got it!"

Persistence in this case has really paid off. Harry (not his real name) calls it his "new way of life," and tells folks that they need to look at tapping like brushing their teeth or eating. "Just do it with the same regularity that you do those things, or even more frequently!"

We began working together intensely about 4 months ago. We continue to spend a couple of hours a week together in session, and he taps no less than three or four times a day. When he grows tired of tapping, he uses the Touch and Breathe Technique or imagines tapping in his mind.

A brief background: At the age of 10, he fell 25 feet down a hay shoot onto a concrete pad, landing on his tailbone. Multiple accidents over the years added to the challenges and pain. He has been through 16 major operations, for his back, neck, and even cancer. He has so much metal in his body that he sets off radar detectors. In addition to suffering multiple major emotional traumas, several years ago he was diagnosed with multiple sclerosis.

As the result of all this, over the years, Harry says he has taken just about every prescription drug on the market for pain (including morphine), and even became addicted to some. The addictions were severe enough that he was forced to enter treatment centers. On occasion he could walk from his home to the mailbox and back without crutches. He couldn't ride in a vehicle for more than 10 miles without excruciating pain and discomfort.

He is now off all pain meds. All multiple sclerosis symptoms, arthritis, and scar tissue pain have vanished, and pain is rarely an issue. When we began, his pain levels, on a 0–10 scale, were generally between 8 and 9 on a daily basis.

An interesting point to make is that as a result of the work we have been doing together, if he begins to experience pain, he now sees a direct connection to someone in his life creating a disruption or aggravation. He immediately taps on the situation and the pain. He affectionately refers to his "aha" point, as his "ha ha" point, because it works so quickly for him he gets a giggle out of it!

Harry attended a workshop I did last year wherein he experienced a great deal of relief from his pain. Unfortunately, after a few e-mails and phone calls, he ceased communication and stopped tapping—this, after going through a subsequent operation, having less difficulty with anesthesia, and recovering more quickly than he said he had ever experienced.

I took it upon myself to reconnect one way or the other (must be the Sagittarian in me!). The night before I called, he and his wife had prayed together because all hope was gone. He was ready to try suicide, once again. He didn't share this with me until we had worked together for a few weeks.

During our first few sessions, he was amazed to see his pain levels drop when we were only addressing the emotional issues and traumatic events. There were tons of them, many of which he was sure he had cleared or had "gotten over" years ago. There were many issues dealing with anger, guilt, and the need to forgive himself and others. We found that adding "forgiveness" to segments of the work we were doing was bringing such rapid improvement, we began adding it as a tail-ender to everything. Another tail-ender used frequently was "without judgment."

Some of the language/issues:

Even though I am sad and angry because I can't play with my grandchildren...

Even though I feel I should be able to do better for my wife, this is unfair to her and she deserves better...

Even though I feel like a failure...

Even though I am stuck taking care of the "IB" (short for insensitive b_____, referring to Mom) because my siblings don't give a hoot and refuse to help...

We also addressed all the physical symptoms, diagnoses, and accompanying fears one by one. A few of the phrases we worked with:

Even though I have been diagnosed with MS, I refuse to accept this disease, I choose to be healthy and strong.

Even though I have this pain and weakness in my legs, I choose to be pain free and strong; I am safe, I am free to be me.

("I am safe, I am free to be me" is a phrase we use quite frequently. As he gained strength, we were able to test with him doing knee bends, unassisted.)

Even though they have told me there is no cure for MS, I bless it and let it go; I choose to be MS free.

Even though I have all this discomfort that feels like a tight headband...

Even though I am afraid everyone will think I am a fraud and a phony when I let go of my wheelchair and crutches...

Even though I fear I may not be able to survive financially if I recover...

Even though I somehow enjoy the attention my condition brings me, I'd rather be able to function fully and under my own steam.

Even though I am afraid the symptoms and pain will return...

Even though I am not sure these treatments will hold...

There were days and times when the emotional intensity seemed almost too much for Harry, but we worked through it, with his insistence that he was ready to offload anything keeping him from healing.

Success: Recently, Harry assisted the Humane Society by driving 136 miles back and forth to the airport with animals, in conjunction with an emergency evacuation for a hurricane. The following day, he worked a shift that exceeded 24 hours, doing everything from building animal crates, moving crates, and loading and unloading caged animals to driving trucks. The following day, he said the only thing that "hurt a little" were his feet. His wife, 8 years his junior, decided to assist, but complained after hour 20 that she couldn't keep up with him!

After 42 years of being in pain, he says it is like having a new life. Harry says he used to dread seeing the sun come up in the morning—"Must I deal with yet another day?" Now, he says he looks forward to every day! "For the first time I can remember there is a spring in my step. Come to think of it, I don't ever remember having a spring in my step!"

A few days after confessing to me about his 24-plus hour day, he did jumping jacks for me as he was leaving our session.

After being on disability for 24 years (yes, I said and meant 24 years), Harry began working a full-time job—not a desk job but one that requires physical effort most of the day. He continues to tap on a daily basis, no less than three or four times a day, and we still work together a couple of hours a week. His wife is still whining that she can't keep up with him. When they get home at night, she is ready to rest and relax while he is still full of energy! Yes, we are working on getting her into persistent tapping as well!

I would encourage everyone to persist, regardless of how hopeless a situation may seem or feel. Harry is a perfect example of what can happen if you just hang in there.

Follow-up, including setbacks, shake-ups, and renewed spirit: It has been about 3 months since I shared the story of Harry and his remarkable progress. I am pleased to report that he is doing great. However, life threw him more than a few curve balls that caused some brief, but frightening and intense setbacks. I feel it is important to share this information, so that those of you working through or with challenging and complex situations might feel encouraged. With challenging cases, setbacks sometimes occur. In spite of this, persistence pays off!

Overjoyed by his newfound freedom, we actually had to tap on *"Even though my newfound freedom has made me forget to use common sense…"* He found himself working to the point of exhaustion on a daily basis, trying to accomplish tasks in a day or two that would reasonably require three or four. I discovered this when I began to explore a new complaint related to "low energy." Another element that popped up was an underlying feeling: "This is too good to be true, my symptoms might return, so I best enjoy this while it lasts." Needless to say, we attacked it with great vigor!

Since things seemed to be rolling along great, we decided to see what we might be able to do in the hearing department. Previous testing indicated 75% impairment in one ear and 80% in the other. Currently, he wears a hearing aid in each ear. The onset of this challenge took place around the age of 7 or 8. While in the care of a disgruntled older sibling, the sibling walked up behind him and popped him up both sides of his head, with the flat of his hands. This resulted in a broken eardrum. Many visits to the doctor's office were required due to ongoing infections and various other ear problems. The doctor continually emphasized the fact that things would only get worse. In addition, family members constantly reminded him: "Nerve deafness runs in the family."

We started by making a list of all the "advantages" of deafness. The list included specific people as well as things he simply wanted to tune out. From there, we went on to the associated "whys" and related events. Another interesting component was determining how much of the challenge encompassed "listening vs. hearing."

As the session progressed, more than once he asked me, "Are you talking louder than usual?" Soon, he was turning his hearing aids down.

I checked in with him late in the day to see how our work was holding. When I asked how the balance of the day went, he replied, "Loud!"

In our next session, Harry was a little frustrated because his hearing improvement seemed to be inconsistent, even though every time it increased, it seemed to be at a higher level. He had made so much rapid progress with his other challenges that he had little patience and wanted immediate and complete results. Yes, we tapped on that as well.

After roughly three sessions and his working on his own between sessions, he was experiencing an appreciable difference. He said he could now "hear inside," referring to the ability to now hear his own voice. He was also beginning to feel vibrations in his face, just at the front of both ears.

A very happy camper, working full time, still tapping daily, and simply loving his "new life," situations arose that caused some symptoms to begin to return. In a week's time, he suffered the betrayal of a son and various multiple major emotional upsets. He was truly on the edge when he came to see me, and his hearing was the last thing he wanted to focus on.

We worked for about 2 hours and, at the end of the session, he was all smiles, symptom free, and back to loving his "new life." Of major interest—during this session we never specifically addressed his physical symptoms.

So now, everybody is happy and once again, life is good. Right? Well, not for long!

Around the holidays, I was out of town for a couple of weeks. While I was away, new disruptions and challenges popped up for Harry on both a physical and emotional level. It seemed that Murphy's Law overshadowed everything. Every day on his way home from work, his physical symptoms would intensify, worsening as the evening wore on. Much to my dismay, all this left Harry in such a state of despair he was actually ready to throw in the towel and go back on disability.

So we rolled up our sleeves and went for it. The good news is that after another intense 2-hour session, he informed me he felt renewed, refreshed, and ready to charge forward and live life to its fullest. Not a trace of wanting to give up remained and the physical symptoms were gone. Once again, during this session we never specifically addressed the physical symptoms.

Some side benefits have popped up as well. Without us specifically addressing his vision in our tapping sessions, his latest eye exam revealed improved vision. He has also been able to eliminate the breathing treatments that were once required at least once a day.

We did work specifically on his annual bout with bronchitis. Every year previous, antibiotics were required. This year, we cleared it with EFT. He says this is the first year he can remember when he hasn't been forced to take antibiotics.

In spite of the interruptions related to working on his hearing, he feels he has already experienced a 15 to 20% improvement. Now back on track, we will see how the progress goes.

One thing I would like to clarify here. I believe that addressing the physical symptoms has great value and benefit. I do so on a regular basis. However, when glaring emotional components are properly addressed, the physical symptoms usually will simply vanish.

The moral of the story is: Keep the faith! Don't despair when symptoms return, be they emotional or physical. The road to recovery can have its bumps, but with persistence we can overcome. When progress seems slow or things seem to be going backward, forge on. It is simply part of the process.

❈ ❈ ❈

The Core Issues in 8 Years of Back Pain: Anger and Forgiveness

By Karen Brodie, EFT INT-1

"Stacy" came to me because she had chronic low back pain. The pain had started after she had been in an auto accident 8 years earlier. At the time of the accident, she had been pregnant with her first child. The details of the accident were that she had been in the middle of an intersection waiting for traffic to clear so she could turn left. As she waited, looking forward and to the left, a car coming from the right rammed into her car without warning. The impact wrenched her back and gave her a soft-tissue injury. Although she and her husband had been extremely concerned about their unborn baby, the pregnancy had progressed normally and their baby girl was born without a hitch later that month.

Other than her chronic back pain, Stacy said that she had a great life. She was married with two young daughters and found a lot of meaning in her work as a wife and mother. She and her family had many close ties in the community to their friends, extended families, and church congregation. Her doctors had given up long ago on finding the cause of her pain, as they could find no medical reason for it, so she was exploring other means of healing. Chiropractic care gave her temporary relief, but she was hoping for something permanent.

Stacy said that, although the accident had been upsetting, it hadn't been traumatic, and it had been so long ago that she was getting fuzzy on many of the details. When I asked her to think about the accident and rate her present-day intensity around it, she gave it a "2 or 3" on the SUD scale. When I asked her to rate the pain in her back, however, she gave it a 7. Since the accident had happened so long ago, and her back was hurting right then, we focused our work on the pain in her back.

I asked Stacy to describe the pain, and she said it felt like a dull ache that was situated to the right of her spine. It was shaped like a ball about 4 inches in diameter. It was in the lower right quadrant of her back and was black and dense.

We did several rounds of EFT using her description. We started with:

> *Even though I have this low back pain to the right of my spine, I totally and completely love and accept myself.*

We tapped on all the points, including the finger points and the 9 Gamut, and then I asked her for the SUD measurement for her back pain. It was "still a 7, or maybe a 6."

We then used several other affirmations, such as:

> *Even though my lower back is hurting right now...*

> *Even though I have had this pain for so many years, off and on, and I just want to be free of it...*

> *Even though I have this black ball of pain in my right lower back...*

None of the tapping got her SUD level below a 5, so I asked her to think back to the day of the accident. I then asked her what, after all these years, stood out for her the most about that day. After sitting quietly for a moment, Stacy said hesitantly that it was the fact that the man who hit her had been willing to jeopardize her safety and the safety of the other people on the road in order to try to be on time to an appointment when he was running late.

We did a few more rounds of EFT using the Setup phrases:

> *Even though the man who hit me put being on time ahead of my safety...*

> *Even though I have had years of back pain just because the man who hit me was driving carelessly because he was running late...*

Even though the man who hit me has caused me a lot of pain over the years, I'm willing to forgive him so that I can get on with my life and let go of this pain.

At this point, Stacy burst into tears. She said that she thought she had forgiven the man a long time ago, but she was feeling angry all over again.

We did a few rounds on her still feeling angry. Her SUD level about feeling angry quickly dropped to 0, but when we were finished with that tapping and I asked her if her back was still hurting, she said it was. It had dropped to a 4, but it still hurt.

I then asked her how she was feeling emotionally. She said she felt better, but that she was feeling disappointed with herself now that she realized she had not really forgiven the man who had hit her until now. She felt that she shouldn't have held on to her judgment and resentment toward him for so long, considering the fact that, in the end, her baby had been fine, and that the accident had happened so long ago. Now she was blaming herself.

We talked a little bit about forgiveness. In my work as an EFT practitioner, I find that, for my clients, sometimes self-forgiveness is the biggest challenge of all.

I asked Stacy if she could think of any reason not to forgive herself for having held on to her resentment for so long and, after a moment's thought, she said no. I know from my EFT work and from my own life that forgiveness, when we have felt deeply wounded, can take a lot of time, energy, and persistence to achieve and I felt a lot of empathy toward Stacy in that moment. I suggested to her that now that she had finally forgiven the man who had hit her, she was in a perfect position to put everything related to the accident behind her; it wouldn't necessarily serve her if she switched the grudge over to herself. After some more thought, she said she was willing to let it all go, but she wasn't sure if she could. We did another round with the Setup Statement:

> *Even though I stayed resentful toward the man who hit me for over 8 years, I am willing to forgive myself for judging him and staying angry for this long. I acknowledge that I was doing the best I could.*

We tapped on all the points and included a 9 gamut as well. After we finished that round of tapping, I asked Stacy how her back was feeling. She said the pain was gone, except for some tightness and residual soreness. We ended the session on that note, as we had been going for an hour and a half, and I felt that we had accomplished all that we were going to in one sitting.

Three weeks later I heard from Stacy. I was very happy to hear her say that by the morning after the day of our appointment, the soreness and tightness in her back had completely disappeared, and had not come back.

❧ ❧ ❧

Quick Start

Now it's time for your first experience of EFT. It's going to take you less than 2 minutes. I'm going to keep it as simple as possible, and I'm also going to give you a practical tool to measure whether or not EFT is working for you. I'd like you to close your eyes and tune in to the area of maximum pain in your back. How bad is it? Let's rate the severity on a scale from 0 to 10. Zero indicates no pain whatsoever. Ten indicates the worst pain possible. In EFT, we call this rating level your SUD or subjective units of distress score (Wolpe, 1958). Write down your SUD score here:

SUD Before EFT _____

See the illustration to locate the first tapping point on the side of your hand. We call this the Karate Chop point.

The Karate Chop (KC) Point

Lightly but firmly, tap there with the fingertips of the other hand while repeating this phrase: *"Even though I have this back pain, I deeply and completely accept myself."* You don't have to believe this, since EFT is not dependent on your level of belief. Simply say the words.

Keep tapping, and repeat that phrase three times.

Then tap on the points in the following illustration (proceeding from top to bottom, beginning with the eyebrow point) with two fingers of either hand 7 to 10 times, on either side of the body, while repeating the phrase "back pain."

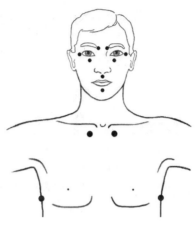

Tapping Sequence Points

After tapping on all these points, tune in to your back again. Write down your new SUD level here:

SUD After First EFT Sequence _____

The chances are good that your SUD level is much lower than it was before. It may not be at a 0 yet, however, so let's apply EFT once more. While tapping your Karate Chop point, say, *"Even though I still have some of this back pain, I deeply and completely accept myself."* Repeat this two more times while tapping that same point. Then, repeat the phrase "back pain" while tapping on every point with two fingertips. Really tune in to your back pain while you do this.

When you're finished, write down your new SUD level:

SUD After Second EFT Sequence _____

The likelihood is that your pain is now much lower than before. Perhaps it's even gone. If it's not entirely gone, no problem, because you've just tried the most elementary form of EFT.

As you read this book and improve your skills with EFT, you'll get better and better at applying it. If you're like most people who do this simple and quick exercise, you're probably quite surprised by how fast your pain diminished. This can encourage you to read further, and start to unlock the many deep-healing benefits of EFT.

Your Next Steps

In Chapter 1, you'll hear from two medical doctors who use EFT. You'll also learn about the science behind EFT. Chapter 2 walks you through EFT's Basic Recipe, after which you'll know the fundamentals of EFT. After that, you can dip into the book to see how other people just like you have used EFT, and be inspired by their stories.

Once you've reduced or eliminated your back pain, you'll want to apply EFT to other areas of your life. I recommend you read *The EFT Manual* (Church, 2013) and any other relevant books in this series. Please write to us and tell us how you're doing with EFT (SubmitStory. EFTuniverse.com). Your story can encourage many other people to persist with their healing journey.

I also strongly recommend taking a Clinical EFT workshop. Most of these are taught conveniently on weekends. A workshop will give you an excellent grasp of EFT's fundamentals as you learn the ropes from expert instructors. I also recommend you work with an EFT practitioner. Try out a few different practitioners certified in Clinical EFT till you find one with whom you click. Your practitioner can help you with problems you can't solve on your own. Together with your doctor, nurse, and therapist, your EFT practitioner can be a key member of your health team.

The bottom line of this book is that you don't have to suffer from ongoing back pain the way you do now. You no longer have to dread the next episode of pain, or accept the limitations to your lifestyle and livelihood that pain imposes. You might tap and become pain free. Or like me, you might have minimal and infrequent pain, reducing its effects on your life to a manageable level. Whatever your level of success, I invite you to take a deep dive into the world of EFT and explore the furthest reaches of its potential to improve your life.

Resources

Clinical EFT: ClinicalEFT.com

EFT for First Aid: TraumaTap.com

Healthcare Workers Study:
    HealthCareWorkers.EFTUniverse.com

Practitioners: Practitioners.EFTUniverse.com

Research: Research.EFTUniverse.com

Submit Your EFT Story to Archives:
    SubmitStory.EFTUniverse.com

Weight Loss: WeightLoss.EFTUniverse.com

Weight Loss Online Course: NaturallyThinYou.com

About Back Pain

Your back hurts, and you're not alone. At least 80% of all Americans suffer from back pain at some point in their lives, nearly 10% suffer from moderate to severe chronic pain, and an estimated 70 million are experiencing significant back pain right now, as you read this. Next to the common cold and upper respiratory infections, back pain is the leading cause of missed work days. Every year 200,000 Americans undergo spinal surgery in an effort to eliminate pain. In the United States alone, back pain costs almost 100 billion dollars per year in medical expenses. Back pain can turn strong people into invalids, destroy careers, wreck marriages, and cause a host of other problems.

According to medical experts, most cases of back pain are mechanical or nonorganic, which means that they are not caused by illnesses such as inflammatory arthritis, infection, fractures, cancer, kidney stones, kidney disease, blood clots, or bone loss. Back pain can be a symptom of these and other diseases, but in most cases it is blamed on sprained ligaments, strained muscles, ruptured discs, irritated joints, repetitive motion injuries, slips, falls, trauma injuries, obesity, weak stomach muscles, overexertion, poor posture, improper lifting, sitting on a back-pocket wallet or billfold, sleeping on a bed that's too hard or too soft, sleeping next to a bedroom air conditioner, carrying a too-heavy back pack, alternating between sedentary and athletic activities, or simply being out of shape. You don't have to do anything dramatic to experience incapacitating back pain, either. Sometimes all it takes is a single sneeze or simply bending over to pick up a pencil.

Mark Grant, an Australian psychologist who specializes in managing chronic pain, says pain can be caused by muscle tension, changes in circulation, postural imbalances, psychological distress, and neurological damage. "It is also known," he says, "that unrelieved pain is associated with increased metabolic rate, spontaneous excitation of the central nervous system, changes in blood circulation to the brain, and changes in the limbic-hypothalamic system, the region of the brain that regulates emotions"(Grant, 2009).

Acute and Chronic Pain

Acute back pain occurs suddenly. It's new. Chronic back pain is long-standing, permanent, or linked to old injuries.

Jennifer Schneider, MD, a specialist in pain management in Tucson, Arizona, states in her book *Living with Chronic Pain* (2009) that the nervous system is responsible for the two major types of chronic pain.

The first, called nociceptive pain, results from injury to muscles, tendons, ligaments, or internal organs. Undamaged nerve cells respond to a nearby injury by transmitting pain signals to the spinal cord and brain. The resulting pain is usually deep and throbbing, such as the pain from chronic low back problems, osteoarthritis, rheumatoid arthritis, fibromyalgia, headaches, interstitial cystitis, and chronic pelvic pain.

The second type of chronic pain, called neuropathic pain, results from abnormal nerve function or direct nerve damage. Damaged nerve fibers fire spontaneously at the injury site and along the nerve pathway, continuing even after the source of the injury has stopped sending pain messages. This type of pain can be constant or intermittent and is usually described as burning, aching, shooting, or stabbing. It sometimes radiates down the arms or legs. The medical conditions that contribute to neuropathic pain include shingles, diabetic neuropathy, reflex sympathetic dystrophy, phantom limb pain, radiculopathy, spinal stenosis, multiple sclerosis, Parkinson's disease, stroke, and spinal cord injuries.

"This type of pain," writes Dr. Schneider, "tends to involve exaggerated responses to painful stimuli, the spread of pain to areas that were not initially painful, and sensations of pain in response to normally non-painful stimuli, such light touch." It is often worse at night and may involve abnormal sensations such as tingling, pins and needles, or intense itching.

Some chronic pain syndromes involve both types of pain. An example is sciatica, in which a pinched nerve causes back pain that radiates down the leg.

In addition, says Dr. Schneider, the consequences of chronic back pain typically extend well beyond the discomfort caused by pain sensations. Her list of potential physical effects includes poor wound healing, physical weakness, muscle breakdown, decreased movement that can lead to blood clots, shallow breathing and suppressed coughing that increase the risk of pneumonia, sodium and water retention in the kidneys, elevated heart rate and blood pressure, weakened immune system responses, a slowing of digestion and gastrointestinal motility, insomnia, loss of appetite and resulting weight loss, and increasing fatigue.

Those trapped in the vice of chronic back pain know that's only the beginning. As health columnist Jane Brody (2007) states: "The psychological and social consequences of chronic pain can be enormous. Unremitting pain can rob a person of the ability to enjoy life, maintain important relationships, fulfill spousal and parental responsibilities, perform well at a job, or work at all." She further cites economic burdens, which can be severe. "Only about half of patients with chronic pain who undergo comprehensive multidisciplinary pain rehabilitation are able to return to work. As for the notion that chronic pain patients are often malingering—seeking attention and escape from responsibilities—pain specialists say that is nonsense. No one in his right mind—and most patients were in their right minds before the pain began—would trade a fulfilling life for the misery of chronic pain."

There are many medical treatments for acute and chronic back pain. Unfortunately, most of them have potentially adverse side effects and very few are considered cures. Even the most aggressive treatments, such as surgery, can have disappointing results, and the most innovative treatments can be prohibitively expensive, especially for those without adequate health insurance.

Because conventional medicine has such a dismal track record, many back pain sufferers have turned to alternative or complementary treatments such as chiropractic adjustments, acupuncture, acupressure, medicinal herbs, massage, postural alignment techniques, hydrotherapy, hypnosis, therapeutic yoga, core-conditioning exercise, aromatherapy, or other modalities, all of which have brought relief to many. Most of these require repeated treatments, which can be expensive and time consuming. In addition, the treatments don't always work. The pain may never improve, or it may go away and come back, or new injuries may trigger new waves of pain in the same old places.

What Causes Chronic Pain?

To answer that important question, consider the discoveries of John E. Sarno, MD. A professor of rehabilitation medicine at the New York University School of Medicine, Dr. Sarno is the author of three best-selling books about musculoskeletal pain. His book *The Divided Mind: The Epidemic of Mindbody Disorders* (2006) explores the many connections between emotions and health.

To summarize, Dr. Sarno says that your back hurts because you are angry. As soon as you realize that and find a way to release your anger, your back will stop hurting. This is why so many promising treatments for back pain don't work, or they work for a while, but the pain keeps coming back. The underlying cause is still there, says Dr. Sarno—you're still angry—and so your body continues to generate pain.

Though Dr. Sarno's theory is not yet accepted by mainstream medicine, thousands of patients have responded to his treatment, and six highly regarded physicians who use his methods contributed chapters to *The Divided Mind*. Like Dr. Sarno, they believe that it is only sensible to treat the emotional factors that cause back pain and the physical symptoms of other chronic health conditions.

Larry Burk, MD, is a radiologist, a physician specializing in X-rays. He has found a divergence between what shows up on scans and the levels of pain and other symptoms that patients report. Here are some of his observations about the link between pain and emotions.

Pain and Emotions
by Larry Burk, MD

It is instructive to note that many ailments that seem to have an underlying anatomical cause may also have a deeper emotional root as well. As a radiologist, I am acutely aware of this situation since there are many scientific studies of MRI (magnetic resonance imaging) indicating that a surprising number of people with no symptoms whatsoever have rather dramatic abnormalities on scans obtained on a volunteer basis for research purposes. Equally puzzling, there are many patients with severe debilitating pain from conditions such as fibromy-algia who have no abnormalities on any MRI scans.

David G. Borenstein, MD, and colleagues (2001) published the results of their research into the predictive value of MRI scans regarding back pain. In their study, 67 asymptomatic individuals with no history of back pain underwent MRI of the lumbar spine. The scans revealed that 21 subjects (31%) had an identifiable abnormality of a disc or of the spinal canal. The findings on MRI scans were not predictive of the development or duration of low-back pain.

Similar studies have been reported in asymptomatic volunteers for MRI findings in the cervical and thoracic spine, the shoulder, and the knee. This research calls into question the assumed cause-and-effect relationship between symptoms and anatomical abnormalities. The same issues are raised by the fact that some patients get better when their physical pathology is corrected through surgery, and some do not. In additional research studies on the placebo effect, sham surgery has produced relief of symptoms when nothing but a skin incision was made at the time of the procedure. All of this information lends support to the concept that deeper emotional issues are at the root, which can be addressed with EFT.

✳ ✳ ✳

To support the theory that pain is caused by anger and other negative emotions, here are some observations from Eric Robins, MD, a Los Angeles physician and EFT practitioner.

Pain and Anger

by Eric Robins, MD

For decades, John Sarno, MD, has seen the worst chronic pain patients in the world. Most lived with severe pain in the neck, back, shoulder, or buttocks for 10 to 30 years. Most received multiple epidural injections, one or more surgeries, and years of physical therapy. They all had terrible mechanisms of action, such as a forklift truck falling on them or a 747 jet rolling over them, and all their X-rays looked like the "Elephant Man." They all had a good reason for their pain.

Yet even with this challenging collection of patients, Dr. Sarno has a 70% cure rate with regard to both pain and function, and an additional 15% of his patients are much improved, typically 40% to 80% better. He has had these results with about 12,000 patients.

Typically when a pain patient goes to a physician for help, the doctor orders an MRI scan, which invariably shows some sort of anatomical abnormality like a slipped disc. The doctor concludes that the disc is causing the pain and prescribes symptom-suppressing drugs or therapies. Unfortunately, this approach usually has poor long-term results. The pain may disappear for a while, but it soon comes back, often worse than before.

Dr. Sarno looked at the medical literature and found an interesting study in the *New England Journal of Medicine*. It showed that if you do MRI scans on 100 middle-aged people who have no back pain, 65% will have a slipped disc or spinal stenosis. In other words, these people have conditions that are blamed for most of the world's back pain, yet they experience no pain at all. He began asking himself, "If the disc isn't causing this pain, then what is?"

What he discovered is that his pain patients had chronic tension and spasm of the muscles of the neck, back, shoulder, or buttocks. When a muscle is chronically tensed, the blood can't flow through it, resulting in a relative lack of oxygen, and this is what causes severe pain.

Then Dr. Sarno asked himself, "Why would someone have chronically tensed muscles to begin with?" He realized that many of us grow up learning, on an unconscious level, that it's not okay to feel or express our anger or anxiety.

The problem, of course, is that, as we grow up, we experience many specific events or traumas that elicit anger or anxiety. As these emotions start to emerge, our unconscious mind basically says, "It's not okay or safe to be feeling these things." Then, Dr. Sarno explains, the unconscious mind causes muscles to clamp down and tighten in order to cause a pain that takes our minds off of what we are angry or anxious about.

Almost all of us, including most physicians, believe that pain serves a useful purpose, that it protects us from more serious damage or injury. By contrast, Dr. Sarno quotes Stanley J. Coen of the Columbia University College of Physicians and Surgeons, who first suggested that psychosomatic physical symptoms were most likely a defense against harmful or toxic unconscious emotional phenomena. In other words, physical symptoms such as back pain are a reaction to unconsciously generated feelings that are repressed as a matter of self-preservation, Dr. Sarno discovered that simply becoming aware of these feelings can lead to a cure.

He obtained his amazing results by bringing folks in for two lectures. In the first lecture he'd tell them, "It's not the disc or spinal stenosis or any other anatomic abnormality that's causing your pain. Most people your age who have no pain have a slipped disc or spinal stenosis or other conditions that are normally blamed for back pain. What is causing your pain is chronic tension and spasm of the muscles."

In the second lecture he'd tell them, "Whenever you have pain, I want you to notice what you're angry or anxious about." Dr. Sarno then had his patients write in a journal, enroll in group therapy sessions, or engage in psychotherapy. He reported that about 20% of his patients weren't consciously aware of what they were angry or anxious about, and those patients needed to work with a therapist to get in touch with some repressed or unconscious material.

I explain Dr. Sarno's model whenever I speak to groups because he gets such amazing results, and, of course, the proof is in the pudding. In one of his books, he explains that this emotional model works not just for musculoskeletal pain; it can be used for most chronic or functional illnesses.

Dr. Sarno's discoveries are an important breakthrough, but the methods he recommends to handle emotional issues are archaic compared to the speed and efficiency of EFT. We can expect better and faster results by combining Dr. Sarno's insights with EFT, which is the best and fastest mind-body healing technique in clinical use in the world right now.

※ ※ ※

In his busy clinical practice, Dr. Robins, who is a urologist, teaches EFT to patients whose symptoms don't respond to conventional treatment. He explains to them that we store trauma not only in our minds, but also in different parts of the body, including muscles, bones, and organs. Most patients grasp the idea immediately and offer suggestions as to what event, memory, or problem might be stored in their kidneys or bladder or other problem area. In many cases, Dr. Robins has canceled scheduled surgery or taken patients off prescription drugs because the drugs were no longer needed.

Research: Reduction of Pain with EFT

Several scientific studies have examined the levels of pain in participants before and after EFT. In the study of health care workers discussed in the introduction, the 68% reduction in pain was achieved in a very short time frame (Church & Brooks, 2010). The participants attended one of five daylong EFT workshops and the pain component of the workshop lasted only about 30 minutes. That was enough to produce a two-thirds reduction in pain.

A randomized controlled trial (RCT) conducted at the Red Cross Hospital in Athens, Greece, examined the symptoms of patients who suffered from tension headaches. It found that after the patients learned EFT, the frequency of their headaches dropped by more than half (Bougea et al., 2013). Not only that, but when they did get headaches, these were on average less than half as intense as before, and their other physical symptoms improved as well.

A second RCT compared a group of veterans receiving treatment as usual (TAU) with a second group who received TAU plus six sessions of EFT (Church et al., 2013). Their pain dropped by an average of 41%, even though the focus of their sessions was their high levels of PTSD symptoms and not pain itself (Church, 2014). This supports the proposition embraced by the physicians quoted in this chapter that much of our pain is emotional. The veterans were receiving EFT sessions for the emotional wounds they'd sustained in service, and 86% of them no longer tested positive for PTSD at the end of the study. When their emotional trauma was resolved, their pain disappeared as a side effect.

When most professionals in the medical field talk about side effects, they're referring to the negative side effects of drugs and other allopathic treatments. In EFT, users often notice beneficial side effects, such as increased confidence, better love relationships, improved business performance, and an overall improvement in physical health. When you improve your emotional state and reduce stress, the benefits show up all over your life.

If Dr. Sarno can produce such significant results just by helping people intellectually understand the underlying causes of their pain, and if Dr. Robins can help his patients cure themselves just by demonstrating EFT in a busy clinic, imagine what you can do with a little time and practice using not only basic EFT, but also some of the sophisticated, effective techniques developed by EFT practitioners. If you read this book all the way through, practice all the exercises, and experiment with all the scripts, you'll be well on your way to healing your back and saying goodbye to its pain.

Resources

Clinical EFT: ClinicalEFT.com

Healthcare Workers Study:
    HealthCareWorkers.EFTUniverse.com

Research: Research.EFTUniverse.com

How to Do EFT:
The Basic Recipe

Over the past decade, EFT has been the focus of a great deal of research. This has resulted in more than 20 clinical trials, in which EFT has been demonstrated to reduce a wide variety of symptoms. These include pain, skin rashes, fibromyalgia, depression, anxiety, and post-traumatic stress disorder (PTSD). Most of these studies have used the standardized form of EFT found in *The EFT Manual*. In this chapter, my goal is to show you how to unlock EFT's healing benefits from whatever physical or psychological problems you're facing. I have a passionate interest in relieving human suffering. When you study EFT, you quickly realize how much suffering can be alleviated with the help of this extraordinary healing tool. I'd like to place the full power of that tool in your hands, so that you can live the happiest, healthiest, and most abundant life possible.

If you go on YouTube or do a Google search, you will find thousands of websites and videos about EFT. The quality of the EFT information you'll find through these sources varies widely, however. Certified practitioners trained in EFT provide a small portion of the information. Most of it consists of personal testimonials by untrained enthusiasts. It's great that EFT works to some degree for virtually anyone. To get the most out of EFT and unlock its full potential, however, it's essential that you learn the form of EFT that's been proven in so many clinical trials: Clinical EFT.

Every year in EFT Universe workshops, we get many people who tell us variations of the same story: "I saw a video on YouTube, tapped along, and got amazing results the first few times. Then it seemed to stop working." The reason for this is that a superficial application of EFT can indeed work wonders. To unleash the full power of EFT, however, requires learning the standardized form we call Clinical EFT, which has been validated, over and over again, by high-quality research, and is taught systematically, step by step, by top experts, in EFT workshops.

Why is EFT able to produce beneficial results with so many problems, both psychological and physical? The reason for its effectiveness is that it reduces stress, and stress is a component of many problems. In EFT research on pain, for instance, we find that pain decreases by an average of 68% with EFT (Church & Brooks, 2010). That's an impressive two-thirds drop. Now ask yourself, if EFT can produce a two-thirds drop in pain, why can't it produce a 100% drop? I pondered this question myself, and I asked many therapists and doctors for their theories as to why this might be so.

The consensus is that the two thirds of pain reduced by EFT is due largely to emotional causes, while the remaining one third of the pain has a physical derivation. A man I'll call "John" volunteered for a demonstration at an EFT introductory evening at which I presented. He was on crutches, and told us he had a broken leg as a result of a car accident. On a scale of 0 to 10, with 0 being no pain, and 10 being maximum pain, he rated his pain as an 8. The accident had occurred 2 weeks earlier. My logical scientific brain didn't think EFT would work for John, because his pain was purely physical. I tapped with him anyway. At the end of our session, which lasted less than 15 minutes, his pain was down to a 2. I hadn't tapped on the actual pain with John at all, but rather on all the emotional components of the auto accident.

There were many such components. His wife had urged him to drive to an event, but he didn't want to go and felt resentment toward his wife. That's emotional. He was angry at the driver of the other car. That's emotional. He was mad at himself for abandoning his own needs by driving to an event he didn't want to attend. That's emotional. He was upset that now, as an adult, he was reenacting the abandonment by his mother that he had experienced as a child. That's emotional. He was still hurt by an incident that occurred when he was 5 years old, when his mother was supposed to pick him up from a friend's birthday party and forgot because she was socializing with her friends and drinking. That's emotional.

Do you see the pattern here? We're working on a host of problems that are emotional, yet interwoven with the pain. The physical pain is overlaid with a matrix of emotional issues, like self-neglect, abandonment, anger, and frustration, which are part of the entire fabric of John's life.

The story has a happy ending. After we'd tapped on each of these emotional components of John's pain, the physical pain in his broken leg went down to a 2. That pain rating revealed the extent of the physical component of John's problem. Two of the original eight rating points were physical. The other six points were emotional.

The same is true for the person who's afraid of public speaking, who has a spider phobia, who's suffering from a physical ailment, who's feeling trapped in his job, who's unhappy with her husband, who's in conflict with those around him. That is, all of these problems have a large component of unfinished emotional business from the past. When you neutralize the underlying emotional issues with EFT, what remains is the real problem, which is often far smaller than you imagine.

Though I present at few conferences nowadays because of other demands on my time, I used to present at about 30 medical and psychological conferences each year, speaking about research and teaching EFT. I presented to thousands of medical professionals during that period. One of my favorite sayings was "Don't medicalize emotional problems. And don't emotionalize medical problems." When I would say this to a roomful of physicians, they would nod their heads in unison. The medical profession as a whole is very aware of the emotional component of disease.

If you have a real medical problem, you need good medical care. No ifs, ands, or buts. If you have an emotional problem, you need EFT. Most problems are a mixture of both. That's why I urge you to work on the emotional component with EFT and other safe and non-invasive behavioral methods, and to get the best possible medical care for the physical component of your problem. Talk to your doctor about this; virtually every physician will be supportive of you bolstering your medical treatment with emotional catharsis.

When you feel better emotionally, a host of positive changes also occur in your energy system. When you feel worse, your energy system follows. Several researchers have hooked people up to electroencephalographs (EEGs), and taken EEG readings of the electrical energy in their brains before and after EFT. These studies show that when subjects are asked to recall a traumatic event, their patterns of brain-wave activity change. The brain-wave frequencies associated with stress, and activation of the fight-or-flight response, dominate their EEG readings. After successful treatment, the brain waves shown on their EEG readings are those that characterize relaxation (Lambrou, Pratt, & Chevalier, 2003; Swingle, Pulos, & Swingle, 2004; Diepold & Goldstein, 2008).

Other research has shown similar results from acupuncture (Vickers et al., 2012). The theory behind acupuncture is that our body's energy flows in 12 channels called meridians. When that energy is blocked, physical or psychological distress occurs. The use of acupuncture needles, or acupressure with the fingertips, is believed to release those energy blocks. EFT has you tap with your fingertips on the end points of those meridians; that's why EFT is sometimes referred to as "emotional acupuncture." When your energy is balanced and flowing, whether it's the brain-wave energy picked up by the EEG or the meridian energy described in acupuncture, you feel better. That's another reason why EFT works well for many different kinds of problem.

EFT is rooted in sound science, and this chapter is devoted to showing you how to do Clinical EFT yourself so you can enjoy some of the benefits research has demonstrated. It will introduce you to the basic concepts that amplify the power of EFT, and steer you clear of the most common pitfalls that prevent people from making progress with EFT. The basics of EFT, called the "Basic Recipe," are easy to learn and use. The second half of this chapter shows you how to apply the Basic Recipe for maximum effect and introduces you to all of the key concepts of Clinical EFT.

Testing

EFT doesn't just hope to be effective. We test our results constantly, to determine if the course we're taking is truly making us feel better. The basic scale we use for testing was developed by a famous psychiatrist, Joseph Wolpe, in the 1950s, and measures a person's degree of discomfort on a scale of 0 through 10. Zero indicates no discomfort, and 10 is the maximum possible distress. This scale works equally well for psychological problems such as anxiety and physical problems such as pain.

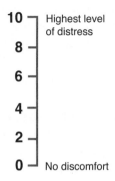

SUD scale (intensity meter)

Dr. Wolpe called this rating the SUD or Subjective Units of Discomfort. It's also sometimes called the Subjective Units of Distress scale. You feel your problem, and give it a number rating on the SUD scale. It's vital to rate your SUD level as it is *right now,* not imagine what it might have been at the time in the past when the problematic event occurred. If you can't quickly identify a number, just take your best guess, and go from there.

I recommend you write down your initial SUD number. It's also worth noting *where in your body* the information on your SUD level is coming from. If you're working on a physical pain such as a headache, where in your head is the ache centered? If you're working on a traumatic emotional event, perhaps a car accident, where in your body is your reference point for your emotional distress? Do you feel it in your belly, your heart, your forehead? Write down the location on which your SUD rating is based.

A variation of the numeric scale is a visual scale. If you're working with a child who does not yet know how to count, for example, you can ask the child to spread his or her hands apart to indicate how big the problem is. Wide-open arms mean big, and hands close together mean small.

Whatever methods you use for testing, each round of EFT tapping usually begins with this type of assessment of the size of the problem. This allows us to determine whether or not our approach is working. After we've tested and written down our SUD level and body location, we move on to EFT's Basic Recipe. It has this name to indicate that EFT consists of certain ingredients, and if you want to be successful, you need to include them, just as you need to include all the ingredients in a recipe for chocolate chip cookies if you want your end product to be tasty.

Many years ago I published a book by Wally Amos. Wally is better known as "Famous Amos" for his brand of chocolate chip cookies. One day I asked Wally, "Where did you get your recipe?" I thought he was going to tell me how he'd experimented with hundreds of variations to find the best possible combination of ingredients. I imagined Wally like Thomas Edison in his laboratory, obsessively combining pinches of this and smidgeons of that, year after year, in order to perfect the flavor of his cookies, the way Edison tried thousands of combinations before discovering the incandescent light bulb.

Wally's offhand response was "I used the recipe on the back of a pack of Toll House chocolate chips." Toll

House is one of the most popular brands, selling millions of packages each year, and the simple recipe is available to everyone. I was astonished, and laughed at how different the reality was from my imaginary picture of Wally as Edison. Yet the message is simple: Don't reinvent the wheel. If it works, it works. Toll House is so popular because their recipe works. Clinical EFT produces such good results because the Basic Recipe works. While a master chef might be experienced enough to produce exquisite variations, a beginner can bake excellent cookies, and get consistently great results, just by following the basic recipe. This chapter is designed to provide you with that simple yet reliable level of knowledge.

EFT's Basic Recipe omits a procedure that was part of the earliest forms of EFT, called the 9 Gamut Procedure. Though the 9 Gamut Procedure has great value for certain conditions, it isn't always necessary, so we leave it out. The version of EFT that includes it is called the Full Basic Recipe (see Appendix A of *The EFT Manual*).

The Setup Statement

The Setup Statement systematically "sets up" the problem you want to work on. Think about arranging dominoes in a line in the game of creating a chain reaction. Before you start the game, you set them up. The object of the game is to knock them down, just as EFT expects to knock down your SUD level, but to start with, you set up the pieces of the problem.

The Setup Statement has its roots in two schools of psychology. One is called cognitive therapy, and the other is called exposure therapy. Cognitive therapy considers the large realm of your cognitions—your thoughts, beliefs, ways of relating to others, and the mental frames through which you perceive the world and your experiences.

Exposure therapy is a successful branch of psychotherapy that vividly exposes you to your negative experiences. Rather than avoiding them, you're confronted by them, with the goal of breaking your conditioned fear response to the event.

We won't go deeper into these two forms of therapy now, but you'll later see how EFT's Setup Statement draws from cognitive and exposure approaches to form a powerful combination with acupressure or tapping.

Psychological Reversal

The term "Psychological Reversal" is taken from energy therapies. It refers to the concept that when your energies are blocked or reversed, you develop symptoms. If you put the batteries into a flashlight backward, with the positive end where the negative should be, the light won't shine. The human body also has a polarity (see illustration). A reversal of normal polarity will block the flow of energy through the body. In acupuncture, the goal of treatment is to remove obstructions, and to allow the free flow of energy through the 12 meridians. If reversal occurs, it impedes the healing process.

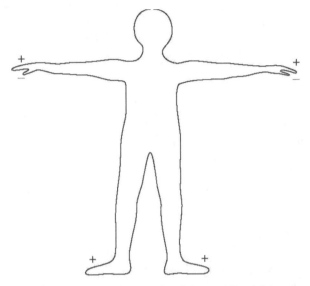

The human body's electrical polarity (adapted from
ACEP Certification Program Manual, 2006)

The way Psychological Reversal shows up in EFT and other energy therapies is as a failure to make progress in resolving the problem. It's especially prevalent in chronic diseases, addictions, and conditions that resist healing. If you run into a person who's desperate to recover, yet who has had no success even with a wide variety of different therapies, the chances are good that you're dealing with Psychological Reversal. One of the first steps of EFT's Basic Recipe is to correct for Psychological Reversal. It only takes a few seconds, so we include this step whether or not Psychological Reversal is present.

EFT's Setup includes stating an affirmation with those elements drawn from cognitive and exposure therapies, while at the same time correcting for Psychological Reversal.

Affirmation

The exposure part of the Setup Statement involves remembering the problem. You expose your mind repeatedly to the memory of the trauma. This is the opposite of what we normally do; we usually want an emotional trauma to fade away. We might engage in behaviors such as dissociation or avoidance so that we don't have to deal with unpleasant memories.

As you gain confidence with EFT, you'll find yourself becoming fearless when it comes to exposure. You'll discover you don't have to remain afraid of old traumatic memories; you have a tool that allows you to reduce their emotional intensity in minutes or even seconds. The usual pattern of running away from a problem is reversed. You feel confident running toward it, knowing that you'll quickly feel better.

The EFT Setup Statement is this:

Even though I have (name of problem), I deeply and completely accept myself.

You insert the name of the problem in the exposure half of the Setup Statement. Examples might be:

Even though I had that dreadful car crash, I deeply and completely accept myself.

Even though I have this migraine headache, I deeply and completely accept myself.

Even though I have this fear of heights, I deeply and completely accept myself.

Even though I have this pain in my knees, I deeply and completely accept myself.

Even though I had my buddy die in my arms in Iraq, I deeply and completely accept myself.

Even though I have this huge craving for whiskey, I deeply and completely accept myself.

Even though I have this fear of spiders, I deeply and completely accept myself.

Even though I have this urge to eat another cookie, I deeply and completely accept myself.

The list of variations is infinite. You can use this Setup Statement for anything that bothers you.

While exposure is represented by the first half of the Setup Statement, before the comma, cognitive work is done by the second half of the statement, the part that deals with self-acceptance. EFT doesn't try to induce you to positive thinking. You don't tell yourself that things will get better, or that you'll improve. You simply express the intention of accepting yourself just the way you are. You accept reality. Gestalt therapist Byron Katie (2002) wrote a book entitled *Loving What Is*, and that's exactly what EFT recommends you do.

The Serenity Prayer uses the same formula of acceptance, with the words, "God grant me the serenity to accept the things I cannot change; courage to change the things I can; and wisdom to know the difference." With EFT you don't try and think positively. You don't try and change your attitude or circumstances; you simply affirm that you accept them. This cognitive frame of accepting what is opens the path to change in a profound way. It's also quite difficult to do this in our culture, which bombards us with positive thinking. Positive thinking actually gets in the way of healing in many cases, while acceptance provides us with a reality-based starting point congruent with our experience. The great 20th-century therapist Carl Rogers, who introduced client-centered therapy, said that the paradox of transformation is that change begins by accepting conditions exactly the way they are (Rogers, 1961).

I recommend that at first you use the Setup Statement exactly as I've taught it here. As you gain confidence, you can experiment with variations. The only requirement is that you include both a self-acceptance statement and exposure to the problem. For instance, you can invert the two halves of the formula, and put cognitive self-acceptance first, followed by exposure. Here are some examples:

I accept myself fully and completely, even with this miserable headache.

I deeply love myself, even though I have nightmares from that terrible car crash.

I hold myself in high esteem, even though I feel such pain from my divorce.

When you're doing EFT with children, you don't need an elaborate Setup Statement. You can have children use very simple self-acceptance phrases, like "I'm okay" or "I'm a great kid." Such a Setup Statement might look like this:

Even though Johnny hit me, I'm okay.

The teacher was mean to me, but I'm still an amazing kid.

You'll be surprised how quickly children respond to EFT. Their SUD levels usually drop so fast that adults have a difficult time accepting the shift. Although we haven't yet done the research to discover why children are so receptive to change, my hypothesis is that their behaviors haven't yet been cemented by years of conditioning. They've not yet woven a thick neural grid in their brains through repetitive thinking and behavior, so they can let go of negative emotions fast.

What do you do if your problem is self-acceptance itself? What if you believe you're unacceptable? What if you have low self-esteem, and the words "I deeply and completely accept myself" sound like a lie?

What EFT suggests you do in such a case is say the words anyway, even if you don't believe them. They will usually have some effect, even if at first you have difficulty with them. As you correct for Psychological Reversal in the way I will show you here, you will soon find yourself shifting from unbelief to belief that you are acceptable. You can say the affirmation aloud or silently. It carries more emotional energy if it is said emphatically or loudly, and imagined vividly.

Secondary Gain

While energy therapies use the term Psychological Reversal to indicate energy blocks to healing, there's an equivalent term drawn from psychology. That term is "secondary gain." It refers to the benefits of being sick. "Why would anyone want to be sick?" you might wonder. There are actually many reasons for keeping a mental or physical problem firmly in place.

Consider the case of a veteran with PTSD. He's suffering from flashbacks of scenes from Afghanistan where he witnessed death and suffering. He has nightmares, and never sleeps through the night. He's so disturbed that he cannot hold down a job or keep a relationship intact for long. Why would such a person not want to get better, considering the damage PTSD is doing to his life?

The reason might be that he's getting a disability check each month as a result of his condition. His income is dependent on having PTSD, and if he recovers, his main source of livelihood might disappear with it.

Another reason might be that he was deeply wounded by a divorce many years ago. He lost his house and children in the process. He's fearful of getting into another romantic relationship that is likely to end badly. PTSD gives him a reason to not try.

These are obvious examples of secondary gain. When we work with participants in EFT workshops, we uncover a wide variety of subtle reasons that stand in the way of healing. One woman had been trying to lose weight for 5 years and had failed at every diet she tried. Her secondary gain turned out to be freedom from unwanted attention by men.

Another woman, who suffered from fibromyalgia, discovered that her secret benefit from the disease was that she didn't have to visit relatives she didn't like. She had a ready excuse for avoiding social obligations. She also got sympathetic attention from her husband and children for her suffering. If she gave up her painful disease, she might lose a degree of affection from her family and have to resume seeing the relatives she detested.

Just like Psychological Reversal, secondary gain prevents us from making progress on our healing journey. Correcting for these hidden obstacles to success is one of the first elements in EFT's Basic Recipe.

How EFT Corrects for Psychological Reversal

The first tapping point we use in the EFT routine is called the Karate Chop point, because it's located on the fleshy outer portion of the hand, the part used in karate to deliver a blow. EFT has you tap the Karate Chop point with the tips of the four fingers of the opposite hand.

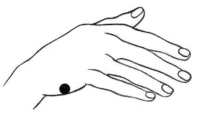

The Karate Chop (KC) Point

Repeat your affirmation emphatically three times while tapping your Karate Chop point. You've now corrected for Psychological Reversal, and set up your energy system for the next part of EFT's Basic Recipe, the Sequence.

The Sequence

Next, you tap on meridian end points in sequence. Tap firmly, but not harshly, with the tips of your first two fingers, about seven times on each point. The exact number is not important; it can be a few more or less than seven. You can tap on either the right or left side of your body, with either your dominant or nondominant hand.

First tap on the meridian endpoints found on the face (see illustration). These are: (1) at the start of the eyebrow, where it joins the bridge of the nose; (2) on the outside edge of the eye socket; (3) on the bony ridge of the eye socket under the pupil; (4) under the nose; and (5) between the lower lip and the chin.

Then tap (6) on one of the collarbone points (see illustration). To locate this point, place a finger in the notch between your collarbones. Move your finger down about an inch and you'll feel a hollow in your breastbone. Now move it to the side about an inch and you'll find a deep hollow below your collarbone. You've now located the collarbone acupressure point.

Finally, tap (7) on the under the arm point, which is about four inches below the armpit (for women, this is where a bra strap crosses).

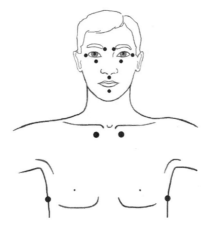

EB, SE, UE, UN, Ch, CB and UA Points

The Reminder Phrase

Earlier, I emphasized the importance of exposure. Exposure therapy has been the subject of much research, which has shown that prolonged exposure to a problem, when coupled with techniques to calm the body, treats traumatic stress effectively. EFT incorporates exposure in the form of a Reminder Phrase. This is a brief phrase that keeps the problem at the front of your mind while you tap on the acupressure points. It keeps your energy system focused on the specific issue you're working on, rather than jumping to other thoughts and feelings. The aim of the Reminder Phrase is to bring the problem vividly into your experience, even though the emotionally triggering situation might not be present now.

For instance, if you have test anxiety, you use the Reminder Phrase to keep you focused on the fear, even though you aren't actually taking a test right now. That gives EFT an opportunity to shift the pattern in the absence of the real problem. You can also use EFT during an actual situation, such as when you're taking an actual test, but most of the time you're working on troublesome memories. The Reminder Phrase keeps you targeted on the problem. An example of a Reminder Phrase for test anxiety might be *"That test"* or *"The test I have to take tomorrow"* or *"That test I failed."* Other examples of Reminder Phrases are:

> *The bee sting*
> *Dad hit me*
> *Friend doesn't respect me*
> *Lawyer's office*
> *Sister told me I was fat*
> *Car crash*
> *This knee pain*

Tap each point while repeating your Reminder Phrase. Then tune in to the problem again, and get a second SUD rating. The chances are good that your SUD score will now be much lower than it was before.

These instructions might seem complicated the first time you read them, but you'll soon find you're able to complete a round of EFT tapping from memory in 1 to 2 minutes.

Let's now summarize the steps of EFT's Basic Recipe:

1. Assess your SUD level.

2. Insert the name of your problem into the Setup Statement: *"Even though I have (this problem), I deeply and completely accept myself."*

3. Tap continuously on the Karate Chop point while repeating the Setup Statement three times.

4. While repeating the Reminder Phrase, tap about seven times on the other seven points.

5. Test your results with a second SUD rating.

Isn't that simple? You now have a tool that, in just a minute or two, can effectively neutralize the emotional sting of old memories, as well as help you get through bad current situations. After a few rounds of tapping, you'll find you've effortlessly memorized the Basic Recipe, and you'll find yourself using it often in your daily life.

If Your SUD Level Doesn't Come Down to 0

Sometimes a single round of tapping brings your SUD score to 0. Sometimes it only brings it down slightly. Your migraine might have been an 8, and after a round of EFT it's a 4. In these cases, we do EFT again. You can adjust your affirmation to acknowledge that a portion of the problem sill remains, for example, *"Even though I still have some of this migraine, I deeply and completely accept myself."* Here are some further examples:

> *Even though I still feel some anger toward my friend for putting me down, I deeply and completely accept myself.*

> *Even though I still have a little twinge of that knee pain, I deeply and completely accept myself.*

Even though the bee sting still smarts slightly, I deeply and completely accept myself.

Even though I'm still harboring some resentment toward my boss, I deeply and completely accept myself.

Even though I'm still somewhat frustrated with my daughter for breaking her agreement, I deeply and completely accept myself.

Even though I'm still upset when I think of being shipped to Iraq, I deeply and completely accept myself.

Adjust the Reminder Phrase accordingly, as in *"some anger still"* or *"remaining frustration"* or *"bit of pain"* or *"somewhat upset."*

EFT for You and Others

You can do EFT on yourself, as you've experienced during these practice rounds. You can also tap on others. Many therapists, life coaches, and other practitioners offer EFT professionally to clients. I'm far more inclined to have clients tap on themselves during EFT sessions, even in the course of a therapy or coaching session. Though the coach can tap on the client, having clients tap on themselves, with some guidance by the coach, puts the power squarely in the clients' hands. Clients are empowered by discovering that they are able to reduce their own emotional distress, and they leave the practitioner's office with a self-help tool at their fingertips any time they need it. In some jurisdictions, it is illegal or unethical for therapists to touch clients at all, and EFT when done only by the client is still effective in these cases.

The Importance of Targeting Specific Events

During EFT workshops, I sometimes write on the board:

The Three Most Important Things About EFT

Then, under that, I write:

Specific Events
Specific Events
Specific Events

It's my way of driving home the point that a focus on specific events is critical to success in EFT. In order to release old patterns of emotion and behavior, it's vital to identify and correct the specific events that gave rise to those problems. When you hear people say, "I tried EFT and it didn't work," the chances are good that they were tapping on generalities, instead of specifics.

An example of a generality is "self-esteem" or "depression" or "performance problems." These aren't specific events. Beneath these generalities is a collection of specific events. The person with low self-esteem might have been coloring a picture at the age of 4 when her mother walked in and criticized her for drawing outside the lines. She might have had another experience of a schoolteacher scolding her for playing with her hair during class in second grade, and a third experience of her first boyfriend deciding to ask another girl to the school dance. Together, those specific events contributed to the global pattern of low self-esteem. The way EFT works is that when the emotional trauma of those individual events is resolved, the whole pattern of low self-esteem can shift. If you tap on the big pattern, and omit the specific events, you're likely to have limited success.

When you think about how a big pattern like low self-esteem is established, this makes sense. It's built up out of many single events. Collectively, they form the whole pattern. The big pattern doesn't spring to life fully formed; it's built up gradually out of many similar experiences. The memories engraved in your brain are of individual events; one disappointing or traumatic memory at a time is encoded in your memory bank. When enough similar memories have accumulated, their commonalities combine to create a common theme like "poor self-esteem." Yet the theme originated as a series of specific events, and that's where EFT can be effectively applied.

You don't have to use EFT on every single event that contributed to the global theme. Usually, once a few of the most disturbing memories have lost their emotional impact, the whole pattern disappears. Memories that are similar lose their impact once the most vivid memories have been neutralized with EFT.

Tapping on global issues is the single most common mistake newcomers make with EFT. Using lists of tapping phrases from a website or a book, or tapping on generalities, is far less effective than tuning in to the events that contributed to your global problem, and tapping on them. If you hear someone say, "EFT doesn't work," the chances are good they've been tapping globally rather than identifying specific events. Don't make this elementary mistake. List the events, one after the other, that stand out most vividly in your mind when you think about the global problem. Tap on each of them, and you'll usually find the global problem diminishing of its own accord. This is called the "generalization effect," and it's one of the key concepts in EFT.

Tapping on Aspects

EFT breaks traumatic events and other problems into smaller pieces called "aspects." The reason for this is that the highest emotional charge is typically found in one small chunk of the event, rather than the entirety of the event. You might need to identify several different aspects, and tap on each of them, before the intensity of the whole event is reduced to a 0.

Here's an example of tapping on aspects, drawn from experience at an EFT workshop I taught. A woman in her late 30s volunteered as a subject. She'd had neck pain and limited range of motion since an automobile accident 6 years before. She could turn her head to the right most of the way but had only a few degrees of movement to the left. The accident had been a minor one, and why she still suffered 6 years later was something of a mystery to her.

I asked her to feel where in her body she felt the most intensity when recalling the accident, and she said it was in her upper chest. I then asked her about the first time she'd ever felt that way, and she said it was when she'd been involved in another auto accident at the age of 8. Her sister had been driving the car. We worked on each aspect of the early accident. The two girls had hit another car head on at low speed while driving around a bend on a country road. One emotionally triggering aspect was the moment she realized that a collision was unavoidable, and we tapped till that lost its force. We tapped on the sound of the crash, another aspect. She had been taken to a neighbor's house, bleeding from a cut on her head, and we tapped on that. We tapped on aspect after aspect. Still, her pain level didn't go down much, and her range of motion didn't improve.

Then she gasped and said, "I just remembered. My sister was only 15 years old. She was underage. That day, I dared her to drive the family car, and we totaled it." Her guilt turned out to be the aspect that held the most emotional charge, and after we tapped on that, her pain disappeared, and she regained full range of motion in her neck. If we'd tapped on the later accident, or failed to uncover all the aspects, we might have thought, "EFT doesn't work."

Aspects can be pains, physical sensations, emotions, images, sounds, tastes, odors, fragments of an event, or beliefs. Make sure you dig deep for all the emotional charge held in each aspect of an event before you move on to the next one. One way of doing this is to check each sensory channel, and ask, "What did you hear/see/taste/touch/smell?" For one person, the burned-rubber smell of skidding tires might be the most terrifying aspect of a car accident. For another, it might be the smell of blood. Yet another person might remember most vividly the sound of the crash or the screams. For another person, the maximum emotional charge might be held in the feeling of terror at the moment of realization that the crash was inevitable. The pain itself might be an aspect. Guilt, or any other emotion, can be an aspect. For traumatic events, it's necessary to tap on each aspect.

Thorough exploration of all the aspects will usually yield a complete neutralization of the memory. If there's still some emotional charge left, the chances are good that you've missed an aspect, so go back and find out what shards of trauma might still be stuck in place.

Finding Core Issues

One of my favorite sayings during EFT workshops is "The problem is never the problem." What I mean by this is that the problem we complain about today usually bothers us only because it resembles an earlier problem. For example, if your spouse being late disturbs you, you may discover by digging deep with EFT that the real reason this behavior triggers you is that your mother didn't meet your needs in early childhood. Your spouse's behavior in the present day resembles, to your brain, the neglect you experienced in early childhood, so you react accordingly. You put a lot of energy into trying to change your spouse when the present-day person is not the source of the problem.

On the EFT Universe website, we have published hundreds of stories in which someone was no longer triggered by a present problem after the emotional charge was removed from a similar childhood event. Nothing changed in the present day, yet the very problem that so vexed a person before now carries zero emotional charge. That's the magic that happens once we neutralize core issues with EFT. Rather than being content with using EFT on surface problems, it's worth developing the skills to find and resolve the core issues that are at the root of the problem.

Here are some questions you might ask in order to identify core issues:

- Does the problem that's bothering you remind you of any events in your childhood? Tune in to your body and feel your feelings. Then travel back in time to the first time in your life you ever felt that same sensation.

- What's the worst similar experience you ever had?

- If you were writing your autobiography, what chapter would you prefer to delete, as though it had never happened to you?

If you can't remember a specific childhood event, simply make up a fictional event in your mind. This kind of guessing usually turns out to be right on target. You're assembling the imagined event out of components of real events, and the imaginary event usually leads back to actual events you can tap on. Even if it doesn't, and you tap on the fictional event, you will usually experience an obvious release of tension.

The Generalization Effect

The generalization effect is a phenomenon you'll notice as you make progress with EFT. As you resolve the emotional sting of specific events, other events with a similar emotional signature also decrease in intensity. I once worked with a man at an EFT workshop whose father had beaten him many times during his childhood. His SUD level on the beatings was a 10. I asked him to recall the worst beating he'd ever suffered. He told me that when he was 8 years old, his father had hit him so hard he had broken the boy's jaw. We tapped together on that terrible beating, and after working on all the aspects, his SUD score dropped to a 0. I asked him for a SUD rating on all the beatings, and his face softened. He said, "My dad got beat by his dad much worse than he beat me. My dad actually did a pretty good job considering how badly he was raised." My client's SUD level on all the beatings dropped considerably after we reduced the intensity of this one beating. That's an example of EFT's generalization effect. When you knock down an important domino, all the other dominos can fall.

This is very reassuring to clients who suffered from many instances of childhood abuse, the way my client at that workshop had suffered. You don't need to work through every single horrible incident. Often, simply collapsing the emotional intensity behind one incident is sufficient to collapse the intensity around similar incidents.

The reason our brains work this way is because of a group of neurons in the emotional center of the brain, the limbic system, called the hippocampus. The hippocampus has the job of comparing one event to the other. Suppose that, as a 5-year-old child in Catholic school, you were beaten by a nun. Forty years later, you can't figure out why you feel uneasy around women wearing outfits that are black and white. The reason for your adult aversion to a black-and-white combination is that the hippocampus associates the colors of the nun's habit with the pain of the beating.

This was a brilliant evolutionary innovation for your ancestors. Perhaps these early humans were attacked by a tiger hiding in the long grass. The tiger's stripes mimicked the patterns of the grass, yet there was something different there. Learning to spot a pattern, judge the differences, and react with fear saved your alert ancestors. They gave birth to their children, who also learned, just a little bit better, how to respond to threats. After thousands of generations, you have a hippocampus at the center of your brain that is genetically engineered to evaluate every message flooding in from your senses, and pick out those associated with the possibility of danger. You see the woman wearing the black-and-white cocktail dress at a party, your hippocampus associates these colors with the nun who beat you, and you have an emotional response.

Yet the opposite is also true. Assume for a moment you're a man who is very shy when confronted with women at cocktail parties. He feels a rush of fear whenever he thinks about talking to an attractive woman dressed in black. He works with an EFT coach on his memories of getting beaten by the nun in Catholic school, and suddenly he finds himself able to talk easily to women at parties. Once the man's hippocampus breaks the connection between beatings and a black dress, it knows, for future reference, that the two phenomena are no longer connected. This is the explanation the latest brain science gives us for the generalization effect (Phelps & LeDoux,

2005). It's been noted in EFT for many years, and it's very comforting for those who've suffered many adverse experiences. You may need to tap on some of them, but you won't have to tap on all of them before the whole group is neutralized. Sometimes, like my client who was beaten repeatedly as a child, if you tap on a big one, the generalization effect reduces the emotional intensity of all similar experiences.

The Movie Technique and Tell the Story Technique

When you take an EFT workshop, the first key technique you learn is the Movie Technique. Why do we place such emphasis on the Movie Technique? The reason is that it combines many of the methods that are key to success with EFT.

The first thing the Movie Technique does is focus you on being specific. EFT is great at eliminating the emotional intensity you feel, as long as it's used on an actual concrete event ("John yelled at me in the meeting") rather than a general statement ("My procrastination").

The Movie Technique has you identify a particular incident that has a big emotional charge for you, and systematically reduce that charge to 0. You picture the event in your mind's eye as though it were a movie, and run through the movie scene by scene.

Whenever you reach a part of the movie that carries a big emotional charge, you stop and perform the EFT sequence. In this way, you reduce the intensity of each of the bad parts of the movie. EFT's related technique, Tell the Story, is done out loud, while the Movie Technique is typically done silently. You can use the Movie Technique with a client without the client ever disclosing what the event was.

Try this with one of your own traumatic life events right now. Think of the event as though it were a scary movie. Make sure it's an event that lasts just a few minutes; if your movie lasts several hours or days, you've probably picked a general pattern. Try again, selecting a different event, till you have a movie that's just a few minutes long.

One example is a man whose general issue is "Distrust of Strangers." We trace it to a particular childhood incident that occurred when the man, whom we'll call David, was 7 years old. His parents moved to a new town, and David found himself walking to a new school through a rough neighborhood. He encountered a group of bullies at school but always managed to avoid them. One day, walking back from school, he saw the bullies walking toward him. He crossed the street, hoping to avoid their attention. He wasn't successful, and he saw them point at him, then change course to intercept him. He knew he was due for a beating. They taunted him and shoved him, and he fell into the gutter. His mouth hit the pavement, and he chipped a tooth. Other kids gathered round and laughed at him, and the bullies moved off. He picked himself up and walked the rest of the way home.

If you were to apply EFT to David's general pattern, "Distrust of Strangers," you'd be tapping generally—and ineffectually. When instead you focus on the specific event, you're homing in on the life events that gave rise to the general pattern. A collection of events like David's beating can combine to create the general pattern.

Now give your movie a title. David might call his movie "The Bullies."

Start thinking about the movie at a point before the traumatic part began. For David, that would be when he was walking home from school, unaware of the events in store for him.

Now run your movie through your mind till the end. The end of the movie is usually a place where the bad events are over. For David, this might be when he picked himself up off the ground, and resumed his walk home.

Now let's add EFT to your movie. Here's the way you do this:

1. Think of the title of your movie. Rate the degree of your emotional distress around just the title, not the movie itself. For instance, on the distress scale of 0 to 10 where 0 is no distress and 10 represents maximum distress, you might be an 8 when you think of the title "The Meeting." Write down your movie title, and your number.

2. Work the movie title into an EFT Setup Statement. It might sound something like this: *"Even though I experienced [insert your movie title here], I deeply and completely accept myself."* Then tap on the EFT acupressure points, while repeating the Setup Statement three times. Your distress level will typically go down. You may have to do EFT several times on the title for it to reach a low number like 0 or 1 or 2.

3. Once the title reaches a low number, think of the "neutral point" before the bad events in the movie began to take place. For David, the neutral point was when he was walking home from school, before the bullies saw him. Once you've identified the neutral point of your own movie, start running the movie through your mind, until you reach a point where the emotional intensity rises. In David's case, the first emotionally intense point was when he saw the bullies.

4. Stop at this point, and assess your intensity number. It might have risen from a 1 to a 7, for instance. Then perform a round of EFT on that first emotional crescendo. For David, it might be, *"Even though I saw the bullies turn toward me, I deeply and completely accept myself."* Use the same kind of statement for your own problem: *"Even though [first emotional crescendo], I deeply and completely accept myself."* Keep tapping till your number drops to 0 or near 0, perhaps a 1 or 2.

5. Now rewind your mental movie to the neutral point, and start running it in your mind again. Stop at the first emotional crescendo. If you sail right through the first one you tapped on, you know you've really and truly resolved that aspect of the memory with EFT. Go on to the next crescendo. For David, this might have been when the bullies shoved him into the gutter. When you've found your second emotional crescendo, then repeat the process: assess your intensity number, do EFT, and keep tapping till your

number is low. Even if your number is only a 3 or 4, stop and do EFT again. Don't push through low-intensity emotional crescendos; since you have the gift of freedom at your fingertips, use it on each part of the movie.

6. Rewind to the neutral point again, and repeat the process.

7. When you can replay the whole movie in your mind, from the neutral point to the end of the movie when your feelings are neutral again, you'll know you've resolved the whole event. You'll have dealt with all the aspects of the traumatic incident.

8. To truly test yourself, run through the movie but exaggerate each sensory channel. Imagine the sights, sounds, smells, tastes, and other aspects of the movie as vividly as you possibly can. If you've been running the movie silently in your mind, speak it out loud. When you cannot possibly make yourself upset, you're sure to have resolved the lingering emotional impact of the event. The effect is usually permanent.

When you work through enough individual movies in this way, the whole general pattern often vanishes. Perhaps David had 40 events that contributed to his distrust of strangers. He might need to do the Movie Technique on all 40, but experience with EFT suggests that when you resolve just a few key events, perhaps 5 or 10 of them, the rest fade in intensity, and the general pattern itself is neutralized.

The Tell the Story Technique is similar to the Movie Technique; as mentioned, the Movie Technique is usually performed silently while Tell the Story is out loud. One great benefit of the Movie Technique done silently is that the client does not have to disclose the nature of the problem. An event might be too triggering, too embarrassing, or too emotionally overwhelming to be spoken aloud. That's no problem with the Movie Technique, which allows EFT to work its magic without the necessity of disclosure on the part of the client. The privacy offered by the Movie Technique makes it very useful for clients who would rather not talk openly about troubling events.

Constricted Breathing

Here's a way to demonstrate how EFT can affect you physically. You can try this yourself right now. It's also often practiced as an onstage demonstration at EFT workshops. You simply take three deep breaths, stretching your lungs as far as they can expand. On the third breath, rate the extent of the expansion of your lungs on a 0 to 10 scale, with 0 being as constricted as possible, and 10 being as expanded as possible. Now perform several rounds of EFT using Setup Statements such as:

Even though my breathing is constricted...

Even though my lungs will only expand to an 8...

Even though I have this physical problem that prevents me breathing deeply...

Now take another deep breath and rate your level of expansion. Usually there's substantial improvement.

Now focus on any emotional contributors to constricted breathing. Use questions like:

- What life events can I associate with breathing problems?
- Are there places in my life where I feel restricted?
- If I simply guess at an emotional reason for my constricted breathing, what might it be?

Now tap on any issues surfaced by these questions. After your intensity is reduced, take another deep breath and rate how far your lungs are now expanding. Even if you were a 10 earlier, you might now find you're an 11 or 14.

The Personal Peace Procedure

The Personal Peace Procedure consists of listing every specific troublesome event in your life and systematically using EFT to tap away the emotional impact of these events. With due diligence, you knock over every negative domino on your emotional playing board and, in so doing, remove significant sources of both emotional and physical ailments. You experience personal peace, which improves your work and home relationships, your health, and every other area of your life.

Tapping on large numbers of events one by one might seem like a daunting task, but we'll show you in the next few paragraphs how you can accomplish it quickly and efficiently. Because of EFT's generalization effect, where tapping on one issue reduces the intensity of similar issues, you'll typically find the process going much faster than you imagined.

Removing the emotional charge from your specific events results in less and less internal conflict. Less internal conflict results, in turn, in greater personal peace and less suffering on all levels—physical, mental, emotional, and spiritual. For many people, the Personal Peace Procedure has led to the complete cessation of lifelong issues that other methods did not resolve. You'll find stories on the EFT Universe website written by people who describe relief from physical maladies like headaches, breathing difficulties, and digestive disorders. You'll read other stories of people who used EFT to help them deal with the stress associated with AIDS, multiple sclerosis, and cancer. Unresolved anger, traumas, guilt, or grief contributes to physical illness, and cannot be medicated away. EFT addresses these emotional contributors to physical disease.

Here's how to do the Personal Peace Procedure:

1. List every specific troublesome event in your life that you can remember. Write them down in a Personal Peace Procedure journal. "Troublesome" means it caused you some form of discomfort. If you listed fewer than 50 events, try harder to remember more. Many people find hundreds. Some bad events you recall may not seem to cause you any current discomfort. List them anyway. The fact that they came to mind suggests they may need resolution. As you list them, give each specific event a title, like it's a short movie, such as: Mom slapped me that time in the car; I stole my brother's baseball cap; I slipped and fell

in front of everybody at the ice skating rink; My third-grade class ridiculed me when I gave that speech; Dad locked me in the toolshed overnight; Mrs. Simmons told me I was dumb.

2. When your list is finished, choose the biggest dominoes on your board, that is, the events that have the most emotional charge for you. Apply EFT to them, one at a time, until the SUD level for each event is 0. You might find yourself laughing about an event that used to bring you to tears; you might find a memory fading. Pay attention to any aspects that arise and treat them as separate dominoes, by tapping for each aspect separately. Make sure you tap on each event until it is resolved. If you find yourself unable to rate the intensity of a bad event on the 0–10 scale, you might be dissociating, or repressing a memory. One solution to this problem is to tap 10 rounds of EFT on every aspect of the event you are able to recall. You might then find the event emerging into clearer focus but without the same high degree of emotional charge.

3. After you have removed the biggest dominoes, pick the next biggest, and work on down the line.

4. If you can, clear at least one of your specific events, preferably three, daily for 3 months. By taking only minutes per day, in 3 months you will have cleared 90 to 270 specific events. You will likely discover that your body feels better, that your threshold for getting upset is much lower,

your relationships have improved, and many of your old issues have disappeared. If you revisit specific events you wrote down in your Personal Peace Procedure journal, you will likely discover that their former intensity has evaporated. Pay attention to improvements in your blood pressure, pulse, and respiratory capacity. EFT often produces subtle but measurable changes in your health, and you may miss them if you aren't looking for them.

5.   After knocking down all your dominoes, you may feel so much better that you're tempted to alter the dosages of medications your doctor has prescribed. Never make any such changes without consulting your physician. Your doctor is your partner in your healing journey. Tell your doctor that you're working on your emotional issues with EFT, since most health care professionals are acutely aware of the contribution that stress makes to disease.

The Personal Peace Procedure does not take the place of EFT training, nor does it take the place of assistance from a qualified EFT practitioner. It is an excellent supplement to EFT workshops and help from EFT practitioners. EFT's resources are designed to work in combination for the most effective healing results.

Is It Working Yet?

Sometimes EFT's benefits are blindingly obvious. In the introductory video on the home page of the EFT

Universe website, you see a TV reporter with a lifelong fear of spiders receiving a tapping session. Afterward, in a dramatic turnaround, she's able to stroke a giant hairy tarantula spider she's holding in the palm of her hand.

Other times, EFT's effects are subtler and you have to pay close attention to spot them. A friend of mine who has had a lifelong fear of driving in high-speed traffic remarked to me recently that her old fear is completely gone. Over the past year, each time she felt anxious about driving, she pulled her car to the side of the road and tapped. It took many trips and much tapping, but subtle changes gradually took effect. Thanks to EFT, she has emotional freedom and drives without fear. She also has another great benefit, in the form of a closer bond with her daughter and baby granddaughter. They live a 2-hour drive away and, previously, her dread of traffic kept her from visiting them. Now she's able to make the drive with joyful anticipation of playing with her granddaughter.

If you seem not to be making progress on a particular problem despite using EFT, look for other positive changes that might be happening in your life. Stress affects every system in the body, and once you relieve it with EFT, you might find improvements in unexpected areas. For instance, when stressed, the capillaries in your digestive system constrict, impeding digestion. Many people with digestive problems report improvement after EFT. Stress also redistributes biological resources away from your reproductive system. You'll find many stories on EFT Universe of people whose sex lives improved dramatically as a by-product of healing emotional issues.

Stress affects your muscular and circulatory systems; many people report that muscle aches and pains disappear after EFT, and their blood circulation improves. Just as stress is pervasive, relaxation is pervasive, and when with EFT we release our emotional bonds, the relaxing effects are felt all over the body. So perhaps your sore knee has only improved slightly, but you're sleeping better, having fewer respiratory problems, and getting along better with your coworkers.

Saying the Right Words

A common misconception is that you have to say just the right words while tapping in order for EFT to be effective. The truth is that focusing on the problem is more important than the exact words you're using. It's the exposure to the troubling issue that directs healing energy to the right place; the words are just a guide.

Many practitioners write down tapping scripts with lists of affirmations you can use. These can be useful. However, your own words are usually able to capture the full intensity of your emotions in a way that is not possible using other people's words. The way you form language is associated with the configuration of the neural network in your brain. You want the neural pathways along which stress signals travel to be very active while you tap. Using your own wording is more likely to awaken that neural pathway fully than using even the most eloquent wording suggested by someone else. By all means use tapping scripts if they're available, to nudge you in the right direction. At the same time, utilize the power of prolonged exposure by focusing your mind completely on your own experience. Your mind and body have a healing wisdom that usually directs healing power toward the place where it is most urgently required.

The Next Steps on Your EFT Journey

Now that you've entered the world of EFT, you'll find it to be a rich and supportive place. On the EFT Universe website, you'll find stories written by thousands of people, from all over the world, describing success with an enormous variety of problems. Locate success stories on your particular problem by using the site's drop-down menu, which lists issues alphabetically: Addictions, ADHD, Anxiety, Depression, and so on. Read these stories for insights on how to apply EFT to your particular case. They'll inspire you in your quest for full healing.

Our certified practitioners are a wonderful resource. They've gone through rigorous training in Clinical EFT and have honed their skills with many clients. Many of them work via telephone or videoconferencing, so if you don't find the perfect practitioner in your geographic area, you can still get expert help with remote sessions. Though EFT is primarily a self-help tool and you can get great results alone, you'll find the insight that comes from an outside observer can often alert you to behavior patterns and solutions you can't find by yourself.

Take an EFT workshop. EFT Universe offers more than a 100 workshops each year, all over the world, and you're likely to find Level 1 and 2 workshops close to you.

You'll make friends, see expert demonstrations, and learn EFT systematically. Each workshop contains eight learning modules, and each module builds on the one before. Fifteen years' experience in training thousands of people in EFT has shown us exactly how people learn EFT competently and quickly, and provided the background knowledge to design these trainings. Read the many testimonials on the website to see how deeply transformational the EFT workshops are.

The EFT Universe newsletter is the medium that keeps the whole EFT world connected. Read the stories published there weekly to stay inspired and to learn about new uses for EFT. Write your own experiences and submit them to the newsletter. Post comments on the EFT Universe Facebook page, and comment on the blogs.

If you'd like to help others access the benefits you have gained from EFT, you might consider volunteering your services. There are dozens of ways to support EFT's growth and progress. You can join a tapping circle, or start one yourself. You can donate to EFT research and humanitarian efforts. You can offer tapping sessions to suffering people through one of EFT's humanitarian projects, like those that have reached thousands in Haiti, Rwanda, and elsewhere. You can let your friends know about EFT.

EFT has reached millions of people worldwide with its healing magic but is still in its infancy. By reading this book and practicing this work, you're joining a healing revolution that has the potential to radically reduce human suffering. Imagine if the benefits you've already experienced could be shared by every child, every sick person, every anxious or stressed person in the world. The trajectory of human history would be very different. I'm committed to helping create this shift however I can, and I invite you to join me and all the other people of goodwill in making this vision of a transformed future a reality.

Resources

Clinical EFT: ClinicalEFT.com

Core Issues and How to Find Them:
CoreIssues.EFTUniverse.com

EFT Community Map:

CommunityMap.EFTUniverse.com

Healthcare Workers Study:
HealthCareWorkers.EFTUniverse.com

Movie Technique:
MovieTechnique.EFTUniverse.com

9 Gamut Procedure: 9Gamut.EFTUniverse.com

Practitioners: Practitioners.EFTUniverse.com

Research: Research.EFTUniverse.com

Tapping Circles: TappingCircles.EFTUniverse.com

Tell the Story Technique:
TelltheStory.EFTUniverse.com

Optional Points
and Refinements

As EFT spread to those with a knowledge of acupuncture, many students and practitioners began to add tapping points. There are hundreds of acupuncture points on the human body, but the most common optional points in EFT circles are the top of the head and points on the wrists and ankles. None of these points are mentioned in *The EFT Manual.* Feel free to experiment in your tapping with any or all of them.

Top of Head. If you run an imaginary string over your head from the top of one ear to the top of the other, the highest point that the string reaches is the top of the head point.

Wrists. Several meridians run through the inside and outside of the wrist. An easy way to stimulate all of the wrist points is to cross your wrists and tap them together (about where your wristwatch would be), inside wrist against inside wrist, inside wrist against outside wrist, and outside wrist against outside wrist. You can also tap on one wrist using the fingers of the other hand held together, patting on the wrist, palm side of the fingers flat against the wrist.

Ankles. Several meridians run through the ankles. The points here are less widely used because they're less convenient, but many people who do EFT include them from time to time. To stimulate these points, simply tap on all sides of the ankle, on either or both legs.

In the reports shared by EFT users in this book and on the EFT website, you'll find other points mentioned, including some that are used in combination. I don't personally use those points or combinations so I won't elaborate on them here. The range of points that produce good results when combined with focused thought illustrate the flexibility and versatility of EFT.

Possible Outcomes

There are five possible outcomes after a full round of EFT.

1. The pain level improves or goes away completely.

2. The location of the pain moves to another part of the body, even if it only moves an inch or two.

3. The quality of the pain changes from, let's say, a sharp pain to a dull ache, or from a throb to a tingle.

4. The pain level increases.

5. Nothing happens.

I'll cover what to do about each of these possibilities in detail, but please note that all of the changes in items 1 through 4 are evidence that EFT is working for you.

1. What do I do if the pain level improves or goes away completely?

If the pain improves but doesn't go to 0, do more EFT rounds until it reaches 0 or plateaus at some improved level. If it plateaus and three or four more EFT rounds don't result in relief, then you can assume that "nothing more will happen" and proceed to item 5.

If the pain goes away completely, you are finished. You have just experienced what we call in EFT a "one-minute wonder." Such immediate results occur frequently, but for those of you who did not experience this, don't worry. It is more common to need further rounds of tapping.

If the pain disappears but resurfaces at another time, this is evidence that more EFT is necessary. It would be a mistake to conclude that EFT didn't work because it obviously did. Our bodies give us many valuable messages (if we are listening) and sometimes a single pain can have several causes. You can try more rounds of standard EFT on the pain and, eventually, the pain may subside permanently. If not, just assume that "nothing more will happen" and proceed to item 5.

2. What do I do if the location of the pain moves to another part of the body, even if it only moves an inch or two?

Any movement of the pain is cause for optimism because it suggests that the original pain has been alleviated in favor of another pain that now gets your attention. It could also mean that the original pain had an emotional cause that was alleviated and the new pain is evidence of a new emotional cause. In either case, start over with EFT at the new location just as though it is a brand new pain.

If the pain moves again, then keep "chasing the pain" until the pain level falls to 0. If you get stuck on a pain that doesn't move or if you don't get relief after three or four diligent rounds of EFT, then assume that "nothing more will happen" and proceed to item 5.

3. What do I do if the quality of the pain changes — for example, from a sharp pain to a dull ache, or from a throb to a tingle?

This is similar to item 2 except the pain changes nature or quality instead of location. Any such quality change is cause for optimism because it suggests that the original pain has been altered. In this case, start over with EFT as though this altered version is a new pain. Keep doing EFT rounds on any future altered pains until the pain level falls to 0. If you get stuck on an altered pain that doesn't move or if you don't get relief on it after three or four diligent rounds of EFT, then assume that "nothing more will happen" and proceed to item 5.

4. What do I do if the pain level increases?

Although it doesn't often happen, I have certainly seen cases in which pain levels increased after one or two rounds of EFT. Other healing modalities refer to the healing response to a therapy in which the individual shows signs of getting worse before getting better. The worsening before the improvement is termed a "healing crisis." Three or four more rounds of EFT will usually move you through the temporary worsening to noticeable relief. If not, or if the relief plateaus at a level above 0, then assume that "nothing more will happen" and proceed to item 5.

5. What do I do if nothing happens?

The high likelihood here is that unresolved emotional issues are major contributors to the pain. This may seem odd to you, especially if physicians have shown you X-rays or other physiological evidence explaining why you have pain, but as discussed previously, pain has both emotional and physical components. There are many cases of chronic, seeming unresolvable pain that have been relieved by applying EFT to trauma, anger, fear, and other emotions. As Dr. Sarno theorizes, the damaging chemicals and muscular tension caused by our negative emotions may be the largest contributor to pain.

So now we need to search for emotional causes to pain and apply EFT to them. Given the variation in emotional histories, this bit of detective work needs to be customized to you. I usually do this by asking questions, such as:

If there was a specific emotional event contributing to this pain, what might it be?

The beauty of this question is that it often points to a vital emotional cause even if the answer you give doesn't seem to at first. Your system has a way of knowing what is going on even when you perceive no realistic link. For example, your back pain may seem to have no connection to the memory of your third-grade teacher ridiculing you in front of the class. That's okay, just use EFT on that memory with a Setup Statement such as:

> *Even though Mrs. Johnson humiliated me in third grade, I deeply and completely accept myself.*

Tap on this and Reminder Phrases for as many rounds as it takes to bring your current emotional intensity on this event down to 0. When completed, you will probably notice relief from your pain. If not, ask the question again and use EFT on the resulting emotional issue. Repeated efforts at this are likely to have two benefits: the emotional events will have lost their sting (probably permanently), and your pain should have faded considerably.

Another good question is:

> *If you could live your life over again, what person or event would you just as soon skip?*

Though this question is more general than the previous one, its answer usually leads to important specific events that need collapsing. For example, if your answer is "My brother Jake," then you can break down your experience with Jake into all the specific events you have had with him that left you feeling angry, frustrated, afraid, and so on.

With these two questions, you can uncover and resolve important issues that limit your life and cause you pain and other symptoms. If you find yourself unable to come up with an answer, use the first guess that comes to mind. If you don't even have a guess, then make one up. Often a made-up issue is as good as or better than a real one. That's because it still came from you and thus isn't totally fictitious. It has your experiences and emotions embedded in it and it can even blend several "forgotten" issues in a useful way.

Touch and Breathe (TAB) Method

Not everyone enjoys or can do the lively tapping that many people who use EFT employ, and in some situations, such as during a business meeting or when dining in public, you may not feel comfortable tapping. An effective alternative is the Touch and Breathe, or TAB, method developed by John Diepold, PhD.

Instead of tapping on each acupoint, simply hold it with a fingertip while breathing in and breathing out. Start by holding your Sore Spot (see the following section) or Karate Chop point, or hold your hands together with Karate Chop points touching, while saying your Setup Statement out loud or to yourself. Then touch and hold each of the EFT acupoints while taking a full breath in and out.

The Sequence takes a bit longer this way, but it can be more comfortable and relaxing, and it works. It's also less conspicuous. Instead of tapping, some people gently massage the acupoints, which is something many of us do instinctively while thinking or concentrating. We may rub or press the upper lip, touch the under the arm point when we cross our arms over our chests, stroke the collarbone, or scratch the top of the head.

To stimulate the hand points, hold each finger of one hand between the thumb and forefinger of your other, "tapping" hand while breathing in and breathing out, or place your fingertips together (index fingers touching, thumbs touching, etc.) and breathe. To activate the wrist points, simply circle your wrist with the opposite hand and hold it while breathing. To access the ankle points, reach down and touch the ankles while breathing.

The Sore Spot

There are two Sore Spots and it doesn't matter which one you use. They are located in the upper left and right portions of the chest and you find them as follows.

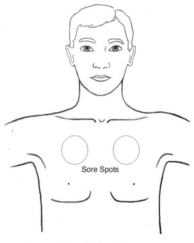

The Sore Spot

Go to the base of the throat about where a man would knot his tie. Poke around in this area and you will find a U-shaped notch at the top of your sternum (breastbone).

From the top of that notch go down 2 or 3 inches toward your navel and then 2 or 3 inches to your left (or right). You should now be in the upper left (or right) portion of your chest. If you press vigorously in that area (within a 2-inch radius), you will find a "sore" spot. This is the place you will need to rub while saying the affirmation.

This spot is usually sore or tender when you rub it vigorously because lymphatic congestion occurs there. When you rub it, you are dispersing that congestion. After a few times of doing this, the congestion is dispersed and the soreness goes away. Then you can rub it with no discomfort whatsoever. The initial soreness should be relatively mild and should not cause undue discomfort. If it does, then lighten up your pressure a little.

If you've had an operation of some kind in that area of the chest or if there's any medical reason why you shouldn't be probing around in that specific area, then switch to the other side. Both sides are equally effective. If you have any doubt about whether you can do this safely, consult your health practitioner before proceeding or tap the Karate Chop point instead.

The 9 Gamut Procedure

The 9 Gamut Procedure is designed to engage parts of the brain involved in the resolution of trauma. It involves eye movements, humming, and counting. It's also designed to engage both the left and right sides of the brain, through counting and music, respectively. Recent research has demonstrated a link between the processing of traumatic memories and the stability of peripheral vision. The eye movements used in the 9 Gamut Procedure take advantage of these discoveries. Clinicians report that it is useful in removing the emotional charge of very early trauma, such as events that occurred in the first few years of life, when there are no conscious memories accessible. The 9 Gamut Procedure is also useful for clearing the intensity of a large number of similar traumatic events simultaneously.

The 9 Gamut Procedure is a 10-second process in which you perform nine "brain-stimulating" actions while tapping continuously on the Gamut point, one of the body's energy points. It has been found, after years of experience, that this routine can add efficiency to EFT and hasten your progress toward emotional freedom, especially when it is sandwiched between two rounds of the Sequence.

As a helpful way to remember how to combine the 9 Gamut Procedure with the Sequence of EFT's Basic Recipe, think of it like a sandwich. The Setup Statement is the preparation for making the sandwich, and the sandwich itself consists of two slices of bread (the Sequence) with the sandwich filling, or middle portion, being the 9 Gamut Procedure.

To do the 9 Gamut Procedure, you must first locate the Gamut point. It is on the back of either hand and is half an inch behind the midpoint between the knuckles at the base of the ring finger and the little finger. If you draw an imaginary line between the knuckles at the base of the ring finger and little finger and consider that line to be the base of an equilateral triangle whose other sides converge to a point (apex) in the direction of the wrist, then the Gamut point would be located at the apex of the triangle. With the index finger of your tapping hand, feel for a small indentation on the back of your tapped hand near the base of the little finger and ring finger. There is just enough room there to tap with the tips of your index and middle fingers of your other hand. That's the Gamut point.

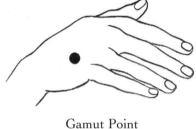

Gamut Point

Next you must perform nine different steps while tapping the Gamut point continuously. These nine steps are:

1. Eyes closed.

2. Eyes open.

3. Eyes down hard right while holding the head steady.

4. Eyes down hard left while holding the head steady.

5. Roll the eyes in a circle as though your nose is at the center of a clock and you are trying to see all the numbers in order.

6. Roll the eyes in a circle in the reverse direction.

7. Hum 2 seconds of a song (I usually suggest "Happy Birthday").

8. Count rapidly from 1 to 5.

9. Hum 2 seconds of a song again.

Note that these nine actions are presented in a certain order and I suggest that you memorize them in the order given. However, you can mix the order up if you wish as long as you do all nine of them and you perform the last three together as a unit. That is, you hum for 2 seconds, then count, and then hum the song again, in that order. Years of experience have proven this to be important. Also, note that for some people humming "Happy Birthday" causes resistance because it brings up memories of unhappy birthdays. In this case, you can either use EFT on those unhappy memories and resolve them or sidestep this issue for now by substituting another song.

One-Minute Wonders

We use the term "one-minute wonder" to describe EFT sessions that produce immediate results, often in people who are trying it for the first time. In those situations, EFT can seem like magic. Sometimes the response is so immediate that there isn't time to complete the Basic Recipe or even an entire tapping sequence.

Here's an example from Jane Beard, who introduced someone to EFT at a dinner party with dramatic results in less than a minute.

Yearlong Nagging Back Pain Gone in 30 Seconds

by Jane Beard

I was at a dinner party with many people I hadn't seen in a while, trying to explain what I am up to now, like studying EFT, and why.

One of them mentioned she'd had a nagging pain in her back for most of this year. We measured her level of intensity and tapped on the Karate Chop point while she twice repeated the Setup Phrase *"Even though I have this nagging pain in my lower back…"*

The third time we spoke the Setup, I added *"…and I'm willing to let this go."* Bingo! The pain left her body as she said the words. We did one round of tapping on the face and torso points and the top of the head (which I have come to call the "yarmulke spot") just for good measure. She was stunned, and so was everyone who saw it happen. Two days later, she was still pain free. That was 14 months ago, and this woman has been completely free from pain the entire time.

❉ ❉ ❉

Following is another case in which the results, although they took longer than a minute, are nonetheless fast and remarkable. The pain, which had lasted for 5 years, disappeared in a few minutes thanks to basic EFT. Note how the author, Sylvia Ross, touches a pain spot before tapping. This helps the client tune in to the specific pain.

Basic EFT Alleviates Long-term Back Pain

by Sylvia Ross

I met with Bonnie, a 58-year-old neighbor who had been diagnosed with chronic fatigue syndrome (CFS) and fibromyalgia 10 years ago. One morning, she couldn't get out of bed and could barely move. She has a history of seizures but had not had any this past year. She is on six different medications, including a type of morphine for pain.

She had not had the opportunity to view the introductory EFT video before her appointment, so that was the first step. The video is great—it makes believers out of first-time clients. Bonnie then gave me an overview of her history, which included mental and physical abuse from her mother, being a workaholic and perfectionist, and the list goes on.

As she told her story, her stress level was rising. I was concerned about her history of seizures so I had her stop and fill out a short intake form listing two symptoms with their levels of intensity on a scale of 0 to 10. The first was upper back pain with a level of intensity of 7 out of 10. The second was lower back pain with a level of intensity of 10 out of 10. She had had pain on and off for 5 years. She listed her basic well-being at a stress level of 6.

We did one round of EFT for pain in her back and I had her gently touch and tap all the points while I rubbed the Gamut point on her right hand. It was all very soft-spoken, as I was concerned about her seizure history, and the Setup Statements were basic:

Even though I have this pain in my back at this intensity and all these memories have added to it, I completely love, accept, and forgive myself, and anyone else.

I asked for a rating on her pain, fully expecting not much movement, but after a look of puzzlement, she said, "It's gone!" Then she yawned at least 10 times. I thought she might fall asleep at the table. At that point it was time for her to go. She talked about how wonderful she felt and said she wanted me to see her son, who has multiple sclerosis, and her husband, who also has back problems. Taking an EFT Chart, she promised to tap at home.

A couple of days later I stopped in to see how she was doing and again she told me how well she felt and her back pain had not returned. The only tapping I did with her that time was for a trigger point on the bottom of her foot that had hurt since major surgery on her ankle after a car accident. I touched the spot to make sure we had located it and then we did one simple round of EFT. Again the pain was gone!

For some reason, my touching the painful area before I do a round of tapping seems to benefit the process. I use it often and have had extremely good results. Usually one or two rounds will clear the pain. It seems to work even better than verbally describing the location in the Setup Phrase, which I also do.

Two-month update: Bonnie's back pain has not returned! I saw her casually in her yard recently and she actually looked surprised when I asked her about her pain. She had had gallbladder surgery a couple of weeks after her original session and had some complications

from the surgery, but she assured me that she had no
back pain.

❧ ❧ ❧

The Acceptance Phrase

The first element of every EFT Setup Statement is
a phrase about the problem. But just as important is the
second part, which is the Acceptance Phrase. The combined statement says that, even though I have this problem, I accept myself. For many EFT students, however,
the Acceptance Phrase is a stumbling block. In a typical
workshop of several hundred people, as many as half
feel uncomfortable saying, "I fully and completely accept
myself." For some, the incongruity is so severe that they
literally can't speak.

EFT can help resolve old emotional issues that contribute to low self-esteem or feelings of guilt or shame,
but for now, if the Acceptance Phrase is a problem for
you, try saying one of the following Setup Statements
while you tap:

*Even though I can't yet fully and completely accept
myself, I would like to someday fully and completely
accept myself.*

*Even though I can't quite fully and completely
accept myself, I'll be okay.*

*Even though it's hard for me to say that I fully and
completely accept myself, I can let go of my fear and do
this work.*

Even though I can't yet accept myself, I can and do acknowledge myself.

If it's still difficult to say that you fully and completely accept yourself, or if it feels untrue, try changing the Setup Statement altogether to something like:

Even though I have this back pain, I would like to feel better.

Even though I have this back pain, I can enjoy life.

Even though I have this back pain, it's going away.

As you experiment with Setup Statements, try different variations. For example, try saying:

Even though I have this back pain, I absolutely do accept myself.

Even though I have this back pain, I love and forgive myself.

Even though I have this back pain, I forgive and accept myself and I forgive anyone and anything that contributed in any way to this pain.

Setup Statements, by the way, can be of any length. While tapping on the Karate Chop point or massaging the Sore Spot, say whatever you like about the problem. You can also talk *to* the problem. Your Setup can last for 5 or 10 minutes or more. The more detailed, specific, colorful, and interesting your Setup, the more likely you are to experience good results. As you read examples of how people have treated back pain with EFT throughout this book, you'll begin to appreciate the important role that imagination and intuition play in the EFT process. Be ready to let your own imagination and intuition work on your behalf as you start tapping.

Here are some recommendations by EFT practitioner Betty Moore-Hafter for softening the delivery of EFT's Acceptance Phrase. Her approach is ideal for those who need to tiptoe into their issues.

Soft Language to Ease the Acceptance Phrase

by Betty Moore-Hafter

As I understand it, the EFT Setup Phrase paves the way for healing by shifting the hard, locked-up energy of Psychological Reversal to the softer energy of self-acceptance. I have found that creative wording can be especially helpful toward this end. Here are some of my favorites:

1. "With kindness and compassion" or "without judgment."

These and similar words contribute an extra dimension of support and care, especially when the issue is a sensitive one. Tears often come to people's eyes as we add these simple words.

> *Even though I feel unworthy, I deeply and completely accept myself with kindness and compassion — it's been hard for me.*

> *Even though I'm so afraid of rejection, I deeply accept myself with gentleness and compassion — I've been hurt a lot.*

Even though I feel guilty for that mistake I made, I totally accept myself without judgment. I'm only human.

It was my friend and EFT colleague Carolyn Lewis who first suggested some of these expressions to me. We trade sessions and, being on the receiving end, I experienced firsthand how good it felt to hear these kind words—and how much emotion they brought up. For me, they went right to the heart. I highly recommend that fellow EFTers trade sessions. You can learn so much by being guided and shar-ing ideas.

2. "I want to bring healing to this."

Some people balk at the words, "I deeply accept myself" and say, "But I don't accept myself! I hate myself for this." One gentle way to proceed is to say:

Even though I don't accept myself, I can accept that this is just where I am right now. And even though I don't accept myself, I want to bring healing to this. I would like to feel better, find more peace, and reach more self-acceptance.

Whenever self-acceptance is difficult, just stating the intent for healing breaks the deadlock of self-rejection. Most people do want to heal and feel better.

3. "The truth is…"

These words can usher in powerful reframes. And when you reframe a situation while tapping, it does shift the energy and things begin to change.

Even though I crave this cigarette, the truth is, cigarettes are making me sick.

Even though I still feel guilty, the truth is, I've done nothing wrong. This is false guilt.

Even though I still feel responsible for my sister, the truth is, she is an adult. She's responsible for herself now.

4. "I'm willing to see it differently."

Sometimes amazing things happen after adding the words "I'm willing to see it differently." One of my clients was convinced that she could never have a child because she might abandon that child the way her father abandoned her. As we tapped through her pain from the father issue, I began adding the phrase, "and I'm willing to see it differently."

Even though my father really hurt me, I love and accept myself, and I'm willing to see it differently.

After several rounds of tapping, she seemed calm and said thoughtfully, "You know, I think my father really did love me in his own way. That's all he was capable of." She felt at peace with it for the first time. And, when I heard from her later, she and her husband were talking about having children. She knew she was not her father and would do it differently. She saw it all differently.

I often tap the EFT points with alternating Reminder Phrases, such as: beginning of eyebrow, "Still feel guilty"; side of eye, "But the truth is…" and so on.

5. "That was then and this is now."

When childhood pain is being healed, people often feel great relief when words like these are added:

Even though when I was 8 years old, I cried alone and no one came, I deeply love and accept my young self. And that was then and this is now. Now I have lots of help and support.

Even though I still feel anxious, afraid that something bad will happen, I deeply accept myself. And even though my child self felt anxious all the time, afraid my father would explode, I love and accept that child self. That was then and this is now. Now I'm safe. I don't need this hypervigilance anymore. I can relax now.

6. "I'm open to the possibility."

"Choice" statements (described in chapter 6) are, of course, very empowering when we are ready for them. But sometimes stating a choice is too much of a stretch. Often the gentlest way to introduce a better choice is simply to bring in the idea of possibility:

Even though I'm full of doubt that I can lose weight, I deeply accept myself and I'm open to the possibility that it may be easier than I think.

Even though I'm stuck in this anger and don't want to let it go, I'm open to the possibility that it would be nice to feel more peaceful about this.

Even though I don't think EFT will work for me, I deeply accept myself and I'm willing to entertain the possibility that maybe EFT will help. I'm ready for some help.

I believe that when we open the door of possibility just a crack, it is enough to set the healing process in motion.

With all of these phrases, you can keep "I deeply and completely accept myself" and add the extra phrase, or you can substitute the phrase. Experiment and see what works for you!

※ ※ ※

Resources

9 Gamut Procedure: 9Gamut.EFTUniverse.com

Practitioners: Practitioners.EFTUniverse.com

Tapping Circles: TappingCircles.EFTUniverse.com

Touch and Breathe: EnergyOfBelief.com

When Your Client Feels Worse:
    ClientFeelsWorse.EFTUniverse.com

Tap While You...

Those who are new to EFT often ask when and how frequently they should practice tapping. The answer is: as often as you like, or better yet, as often as possible. EFT is very flexible and forgiving. The more often you practice, the sooner EFT will become a familiar tool that you can use without effort. The more you use it, the better it works. The more you use it, the more likely you are to remember to use it when you really need it.

Where and When to Tap

I suggest that you start by tapping: as soon as you wake up in the morning, before every meal, and before falling asleep at night. That's five times a day right there. Tap whenever you use the bathroom or take a shower and you'll add a few more times. Some people tap whenever they come to a stop sign or red light. Quite a few tap while they walk. You don't have to do the entire Basic Recipe. Just a few quick taps as time permits will help keep your

ess level low. As soon as you have enough time, follow
) with the complete sequence. Many people tap before,
during, or after they pray or meditate. It is no exaggera-
tion to say that EFT tapping can improve any project or
activity.

One of our EFT success stories is Irene Mitchell,
whose leg was so badly shattered in a car accident that
doctors did not expect her to live. She survived, but they
warned her that she probably wouldn't walk again. She
learned EFT while recuperating at a rehabilitation nursing home, and the first thing she used it for was pain
relief. A few fast rounds of tapping would eliminate the
pain in her leg and hip for as long as 90 minutes, and then
she would tap again. In this way she was able to stop
taking pain medication. She also used EFT to improve
the results of her physical therapy sessions, in some cases
accomplishing in 10 minutes what most people need
weeks to achieve. Thanks to EFT, Irene left the nursing
home several months ahead of schedule and resumed her
active life, which included parasailing on a cruise vacation
and dancing onstage at Disneyland!

When asked how often she tapped, Irene answered,
"At least a hundred times a day. EFT was my pain medication. It got me out of the wheelchair, and it helped me
fix any problem that occurred. I encourage anyone who's
reading this book to use EFT as often as possible. With
EFT's help, your mind and emotions can be powerful
allies in helping you live a pain-free life."

When you're in a hurry, try tapping on a single point,
such as the Karate Chop point, while you focus on your

pain or problem. People have gotten results simply by tapping on the Karate Chop point while reciting a Setup Statement.

Tapping on the EFT acupoints without reciting a Setup Statement or focusing your thoughts on anything specific can be beneficial too, though, obviously, your results are unlikely to be as profound as when you complete the Basic Recipe.

Try tapping to music. This is a popular activity in some EFT workshops. It keeps the group focused and energetic, and it's an easy way to avoid an energy slump in the afternoon. Teaching children to tap to music is a great way to introduce them to EFT. Tap at whatever rhythm feels right. Experiment with classical music, rock, ballads, opera, military marches, movie soundtracks, or whatever you most enjoy.

Tap while you read your e-mail or work at the computer. Tap while you watch TV. Tap while you talk on the phone. Tap while you study; that's an easy way to improve your reading comprehension and recall. Tap right now as you read this page.

If you tap while you describe things that you've seen or experienced, your recollections are more likely to be accurate. In EFT, we use the Tell the Story and Watch the Movie techniques to help people describe or replay difficult events without feeling emotionally overwhelmed. With their emotions under control, they are able to think, remember, and process information more efficiently. EFT practitioners have reported on tapping's calming effect when applied immediately after an accident, tragedy, or disaster.

The following is a suggestion from EFT practitioner Rick Wilkes on another opportunity for tapping. It has special application for those experiencing back pain because it deals with underlying issues easily and automatically, without conscious effort. Some have found that their back pain disappeared completely as a result of following Rick's simple instructions.

The Tap-While-You-Gripe Technique
by Rick Wilkes

Have you ever called a friend just to gripe about everything that's gone wrong in your day? The truth is that when things go wrong, we need to feel that we're not alone. So we turn to trusted friends and family to let off steam and be comforted. It's a natural part of being human. Most of us have been expressing our pain this way since we were very young children.

What I call "griping" is just a way to retell a story with emotional intensity. And there is scientific proof that this can help us. Recent brain studies show that there's an *opportunity* when we relive an experience to have the stored emotions of that experience heal...or become even more intense. As we recall the story and feel the emotions in our body, our brain is making a decision—one that can go either way! Here's how it works.

Let's say the story that we're telling is one in which we feel alone and unsupported. If we tell that story to a friend who is loving, present, kind, and comforting, chances are that our primitive emotional brain will no longer feel alone and unsupported, right? In the process of telling the story, we heal the emotional intensity. That is the ideal outcome.

Yet, how often has it happened to you that in the process of telling and retelling an intense story, explaining about how you were "done wrong" by someone else, you find that after the second or third or fourth retelling that the pain is now more intense than it was right after it happened? That's the risk of sharing our painful experiences with others, whether they are talk professionals or not—unless you are using a technique that consistently allows you to eliminate and then harmonize the emotional intensity. And EFT is just such a technique.

That is why I suggest that you always tap while you gripe. Tap while you complain. Tap every time you tell a story that has negative emotional intensity. Pretty soon, you'll probably notice you have a lot less in your life to gripe about!

Here's how you can get started:

You've had a bad day. You want to feel that there's someone out there that understands you, that cares about you, that takes your side. So you pick up the phone, and you call your best friend. Start tapping... and tap continuously while you talk to her!

(Karate Chop) *Ring...Ring...Hello?*

(Top of Head) *Oh, I'm so glad I reached you.*

(Inside Eyebrow) *I have had such a terrible day!*

(Side of Eye) *I really need someone to talk to.*

(Under Eye) *Do you have a few minutes?*

(Under Nose) *First off, this *&^%$ boss of mine…*

(Then Chin, Collarbone, Under the Arm, Karate Chop, and back to Top of Head, etc.)

The order of the points doesn't matter. The number of taps at each point doesn't matter. You can tap one point that feels good the whole call if you want. You can use the finger points (see Appendix A in *The EFT Manual*). Just tap continuously while you talk. Don't stop!

Why would we do this? We talk to others to feel better, don't we? But there are two approaches to griping and complaining. The first is, alas, the more common. It is to gather people to our side in the upcoming war. We tell a story to make us "right" and the other party "wrong." With this plan, we must build intensity in ourselves and in others while we plan revenge (or a lawsuit, divorce, or other dramatic action designed so we win and the other loses).

The other approach is to want to heal from an emotional pain, and we're mature enough to know that intensifying the fear by making us the "Victims" and others into the "Powerful Forces of True Evil" just creates war inside us, not peace.

We make our healing far more likely if we just tap the acupoints while we express our hurt and our anger and our sadness and our feelings of being out of control. We use what has been human nature since cave folks sat around the fire—the need to tell our story to tribe members to gain their supportive energy—and we use that supportive energy in a new way that is far more likely to result in a sense of peace for all of us.

What I find is that tapping while I gripe and complain shifts my entire perspective. As the noise of the emotional disruption settles down, I am far more likely to hear my intuition guide me to steps that resolve the situation in the best possible way.

Try it for yourself. Tap the acupoints while you are on the phone. No one needs to know that you are tapping. Notice whether there is a change that helps you feel both more peaceful and more empowered. I am confident there will be.

In fact, you may find this so effective that you pick up your phone and tap while you gripe without even calling your friend. Once you get it all out of your system, then you dial...and perhaps have a very different kind of conversation.

☼ ☼ ☼

Can You Do EFT Incorrectly?

EFT is so forgiving and versatile that finding ways in which it doesn't work can be a challenge. In fact, many people who use EFT respond that the only way to do it wrong is not to use it.

That said, it is possible to do an incomplete EFT treatment, that is, not to get to the emotional issues that are underlying the problem you are addressing. This will make more sense as we explore core issues and other advanced concepts in the upcoming chapters. For now, if you combine focused thought and intention with tapping, your efforts will probably produce positive effects, no matter what Setup Statement or modified tapping sequence you use. For example, you can omit the words "Even though" and simply state the problem:

My back hurts.

You can omit the "I completely and fully accept myself" phrase and simply say:

I'm okay.

This, by the way, is how we use EFT with children. A child who's upset can say:

Even though I flunked the math test, I'm a cool kid, I'm okay.

Even though I lost my backpack and I'm mad at myself, I'm still an awesome kid.

You don't have to tap on the EFT acupoints in any specific order. I recommend the Sequence as described because it's easy to remember, but you can also tap as follows:

- Tap from top to bottom.
- Tap from bottom to top.
- Tap on every other point, then tap on the remaining points.
- Tap first on one side of the body, then the other.

- Tap on one side of the body and not the other.
- Tap really fast, at a rate of several taps per second.
- Tap really fast, moving quickly from one point to the next.
- Tap very slowly, at the rate of one tap or less per second.
- Tap very slowly, staying for a full minute or more at each point.
- Tap on a single point and forget about the rest.
- Tap on a photo or drawing of yourself or another person.
- Tap mentally, in your head, without touching the points at all.

If your intention is to treat a specific issue, such as the pain in your lower back, and you combine that intention with any type of acupoint stimulation, you can expect good results.

Other meridian-based therapies use different tapping patterns for different conditions or symptoms, each having its own sequence. These patterns can be difficult to remember, especially in emergencies. EFT's single tapping pattern streamlines the process. By the time you complete three or more rounds of tapping on the EFT acupoints, you've tapped on all of the points in a variety of combinations. The beauty of meridian therapies is that when you stimulate points that you don't need, you don't hurt yourself or cause complications, and when you tap on points that you do need, the process works.

Learning EFT's Full Basic Recipe, including all the finger points and the 9 Gamut Procedure, is worthwhile because these are good tools to have at your disposal should the need arise. For example, when your SUD level does not go down and you've tried all the suggestions offered previously, it is often possible to shift it by doing the Full Basic Recipe. In most cases, however, you will likely get good results without these additional tapping points and methods.

It is helpful to identify your personal EFT acupoint. Most of us, if we pay attention, realize that we're drawn to a certain point, or we notice that every time there is a change in how we feel, it's when we're tapping on the same point. For some, it's the point under the eye or the chin point; for many, it's the Karate Chop point. If you set out to relieve your back pain and you tap on a single acupoint and the pain goes away, you need go no further, unless you want to explore the full array of EFT's health benefits.

How to Tell When EFT Is Working

Did your tapping make a difference? When the problem is pain, the test is simple: Either the pain goes away or it doesn't. If it does, it's probably because EFT successfully lowered your stress while neutralizing emotional issues that contributed to the pain's underlying cause. Pain relief isn't the only indication of EFT's effectiveness, however. Here are some common signs of EFT at work in any tapping session.

- The person sighs. This often happens after a round of tapping and it reflects an energy shift away from stress toward relaxation.

- The person yawns. The yawn might or might not be accompanied by fatigue. Some people have fallen asleep in the middle of their EFT sessions, but even well-rested people yawn during and after tapping. Yawning has been associated with sleepiness, boredom, and (incorrectly) low blood oxygen levels. Behaviorists consider yawning a calming signal, a nonthreatening bit of body language designed to help those nearby relax and feel safe. Recent research suggests that yawning is a way to cool the brain. Whatever its purpose, yawning in an EFT session is an important clue that the tapping is working to lower the individual's stress.

- The person's breathing changes. Most of us breathe shallowly, especially when we're under stress. Longer, slower, deeper breaths are almost always a signal that EFT is working. The calmer you become and the lower your stress, the smoother and more relaxed your breathing.

- The person's voice changes. During an EFT session it's not uncommon for someone's voice to crack, for stress or tension to make the voice actually squeak, or for the person to have trouble talking. Then, after using EFT to lower the stress, the person's voice sounds deeper, rounder, fuller, more confident, stronger, and more vibrant. Speech patterns change, too, going from stumbling and inarticulate to clear, coherent, fluid, and eloquent.

- The person's posture and body language change. People who are depressed, anxious, frightened, or in pain sit, stand, and walk very differently from the way they do when they're comfortable, confident, relaxed, happy, and healthy. In successful EFT sessions, postural changes are often obvious. Instead of sitting hunched, with the head down and a curved spine, most people straighten up, lift their heads, and look at the world around them. Some practitioners describe their clients as blossoming like flowers as their stress level is reduced.

- The person cries. The Tearless Trauma Technique is at the heart of EFT, and it really is possible to work through serious problems without weeping. But in many cases, people do cry. Tears are often a sign of release or relief. Even if the tears are a symptom of discomfort, in which case the Tearless Trauma Technique is used to reduce the discomfort level, the emotional change indicates that EFT is working.

- Sinuses drain. Congested sinuses that suddenly begin to drain reflect an energy shift.

- Facial muscles relax. Actually, muscles all over the body soften, but changes in facial expression, such as from tense and stressed to relaxed and comfortable, are obvious clues. EFT can make such a difference in facial expression that some practitioners call it an instant face-lift. With effective tapping, you may look years younger as well as happier.

- Blood pressure and pulse change. Often people begin an EFT session with an elevated pulse rate or high blood pressure. Successful EFT tapping, even if it's for something unrelated to physical symptoms, can bring both pulse and blood pressure back to normal.

- The person feels hot or cold. A temperature change, such as feeling suddenly hot or cold, is another indication that EFT is working. A small or large area of back pain may feel intensely warm or hot, and the pain may pulse or vibrate. Someone who feels suddenly hot may blush or turn red. Another person might break out in a cold sweat and suddenly feel chilled. All of these physiological changes indicate that EFT is working.

- The person feels vibrating energy. Do enough tapping and your fingers will begin to tingle. When that happens, move your open hands toward each other, moving them closer, further apart, and closer again. If you sense a vibrating energy field or a feeling of resistance that grows stronger as your hands move closer, something is happening energetically.

- A cognitive shift occurs. One minute you're angry and the next you're laughing. One minute the person you're mad at can't do anything right and the next you're making excuses for him. One minute you're convinced that there is only one way, one "right" and "true" way, to look at the situation and the next you realize there are many. As soon as you stop replaying a situation in the same old way and notice something new or different, and as soon as "the principle of the thing" no longer matters the way it did, it's obvious that EFT has done its job.

- The pain moves. This happens so often that we use the phrase "chasing the pain" to describe the appropriate EFT response, which is to tap for the pain's new location. The pain might move a short distance, such as an inch or two, but it's often a longer distance, such as from the left eye to the right side of the forehead or from the right shoulder blade to the center of the spine. In some cases, pain jumps all over the body. For example, you might be tapping for pain in the small of your back and suddenly realize that your back pain has disappeared, but now your right ankle is throbbing. Moving pain is a definite indication that EFT is working.

- The pain gets worse. Ironically, this can be a sign that EFT is working. It often indicates that buried emotional issues are getting close to the surface. By continuing to tap and by approaching the pain and its aspects from a different perspective, your results will probably improve. It's very unusual for pain to get worse and stay worse when you're using EFT, especially when you incorporate the many shortcuts and advanced techniques explained in this book.

- The person is suddenly open to new options. This is an excellent sign because it shows that the person is no longer stuck in an old way of thinking and feeling. Reduced stress supports clear thinking.

You could say that the overall test of whether EFT is working is whether *any* kind of change is taking place.

The more things change, the more apparent it is that there is a shift from stress toward relaxation. Even if you haven't yet achieved the results you hope for, this shift is a very good sign. It is only when nothing happens—the pain stays exactly where it was, your attitude doesn't shift at all, and the whole situation stays stuck—that you may be tempted to conclude that EFT was not effective.

In EFT, so much depends on the art of delivery, the search for core issues, and the examination of different aspects that a sudden breakthrough can turn an unresponsive situation into a success. Many people have experienced this in their tapping. Rather than conclude that EFT didn't work, continue tapping. Sometimes we have to search more diligently for a problem's true emotional cause.

The next chapter will teach you how to conduct this search. As you learn how to identify and address the core issues underlying your back pain, you will be taking your EFT skills to a new level.

Resources

Movie Technique:
MovieTechnique.EFTUniverse.com

9 Gamut Procedure: 9Gamut.EFTUniverse.com

Tapping Circles: TappingCircles.EFTUniverse.com

Tearless Trauma: TearlessTrauma.EFTUniverse.com

Tell the Story Technique:
TelltheStory.EFTUniverse.com

5

Exploring
Underlying Issues

Occasionally, someone uses the basic EFT protocol and gets immediate, lasting results. "One-minute wonders" can and do happen, even with incapacitating back pain. In many cases, however, after EFT reduces or eliminates the pain, it returns. If this happens to you, don't assume that EFT didn't work. EFT worked fine on the problem you treated, but a new aspect of that problem may have presented itself and needs attention or you may need to be more specific in how you are stating the problem. See chapter 2 for guidance on aspects and being specific. In this chapter, we explore underlying issues and how to address them to increase your EFT effectiveness.

Defining the Pain

If you work with an EFT practitioner, you will be asked certain questions, the purpose of which may not be clear to you at first. Be assured, however, that these questions are designed to help you access the specific language that will get to the root of your pain and produce results in your tapping. For example, a practitioner might invite you to use your imagination in describing the nature of your pain, such as imagining what your pain would sound like if it had a sound. Using the imagination is a way to sidestep the conscious mind and access unconscious issues that might contribute to pain. To help improve your receptiveness to these ideas, tap on the EFT acupoints while you read and answer the following questions. The sample answers given are from actual EFT clients and students.

1. **Describe the pain.** Where is it? How big is it? What shape is it? What number do you give it on the 0-to-10 scale?

   It's a rectangular box about the size and shape of a videotape buried deep in my shoulder, and it's a 9 right now.

   It's a flattened oval, the size and shape of a squashed grapefruit. It covers my lower back. I can't move. It's a 10.

   It's three small hard marbles in my upper right hip. When I press against them, the pain is a 6 or 7. When I try to do yoga, it's a 9 or 10.

   It's a heavy wet blanket that covers my spine. It's a pretty constant 5 or 6. I can still walk and move, but it hurts all the time and weighs me down, and I always know it's there.

2. **What color is it?** Is it bright or dull? Glossy or matte? Solid or dappled? Vivid or muted? Neon or pastel? Transparent or opaque? Clear or hazy? Blurry or in focus?

It's bright yellow with orange flecks at the edges like a flame.

It's a deep red-orange.

It's navy blue, like a dark velvet blue.

It's a bright, clearly delineated orange oval surrounded by an indistinct reddish swirling cloud.

It's a grimy dull mustard yellow. It needs a bath.

It's a bright electric neon blue.

It's black. When it lightens up, it's charcoal gray.

3. **What is its texture?** Is it rough or smooth? Hard or soft? Solid or spongy? Does it hold its shape or shift and change?

   It's hard with a rough, grainy surface.

   It's very hard and spiky, with thorns all over.

   It's soft and oozy, like Jell-O. It undulates.

   It's fuzzy.

   It's raspy, like rough sandpaper.

   It's a ball of electricity that shoots lightning bolts down my spine.

   It's thin and sharp like a needle or an ice pick.

4. **Does it make a sound?** Do you hear a noise, a voice, a rustle, a crackle?

   It's a dull, heavy, background roar, like highway traffic.

   It crackles, like a wood fire or like paper burning.

   It's shrill, like a dentist's drill.

I hear a lot of static.

It grates and grinds, making a noise like gravel.

5. **Is the pain steady, or does it pulse or throb?** Is the throbbing intermittent or ongoing? Does the pain come in waves? Does it have a rhythm?

    It's a dull, throbbing, monotonous pain that never stops.

    It comes and goes. When I least expect it, it zaps me hard.

    It's like the tides. It starts in the morning at a low level and rises up all day, then at night it recedes.

    It moves in ripples or waves, starting in my right hip and moving across my back to my left shoulder.

6. **What does the pain remind you of?** One way to get a good answer to this important question is to say, "This pain reminds me of ____" or "This pain makes me think of ____," and wait for your mind to fill in the blank.

    This pain reminds me of being sick when I was a kid and feeling totally helpless.

    This reminds me of the time I painted the house because I couldn't afford to hire anyone and I sprained my back.

    This pain makes me think of how much I hate my job.

    This pain makes me think about my sister-in-law and all the time I had to spend with her planning my niece's wedding. I'm still exhausted.

7. **When did the pain first appear?** What were you doing? What was happening in your life? What is your pain's history?

This pain started the week my brother got arrested.

This pain started right after I found out I was pregnant.

The day I got laid off, I came home from work and tripped on the stairs. I've been hurting ever since.

My back has been in spasms ever since my wife walked out on me.

8. **How does the pain make you feel?** This is another crucial question because EFT is *Emotional* Freedom Techniques, and emotions are an underlying cause, or contributing factor, in most pain, especially chronic pain. Does the pain make you angry, frustrated, upset, sad, depressed, irritated, or confused?

    I feel guilty because I'm impatient with everyone, including the cat.

    Are you kidding? I'm furious! This pain has wrecked my life!

    I get so discouraged. Everything's an effort. Nothing seems to help. Why bother trying?

    I'm worried about everything—my business, the kids, money. All I do is hurt and feel sick about not being able to do anything.

9. **Is there anything else we need to know about this pain?** A good way to address this question is to say, "This pain must be here because _____" or "This pain makes me realize _____."

    This dark gloomy black awful wet blanket of pain must be here because my adjustable rate mortgage is going up again, I may lose the house, and I'm too depressed to think straight.

This bright orange ball of pain in my lower back makes me realize how much I hate living next door to my sister.

This pain makes me realize what a big mistake it was to buy a new truck.

This pain is here to punish me for what I did last summer.

10. **Has your condition been diagnosed by a physician?**
    If so, including this information is another way to be specific. For many, a medical diagnosis complete with official terminology makes the diagnosis "real."

    Even though I was diagnosed with herniated nucleus pulposus lumbar spine at the L5 level...

    Even though I have a C5-C6 cervical herniated disc that is compressing my spinal cord...

    Even though I have degenerative adult scoliosis...

If you don't have a specific diagnosis, you can still take advantage of the effect that medical terminology exerts on you and your emotions. Borrowing from the preceding descriptions of back pain, consider saying:

Even though I have deep, throbbing nociceptive pain resulting from old injuries and involving muscle tension, changes in circulation, postural imbalances, psychological distress, neurological effects, spontaneous excitation of the central nervous system, and changes in my limbic-hypothalamic system...

Even though I have chronic neuropathic pain from nerve damage, resulting in exaggerated responses to painful stimuli and constant or intermittent burning, aching, shooting, or stabbing pain that fires spontaneously at old injury sites and at other locations along the nerve pathway...

As you examine the pain, keep tapping and adding to your description so that your Setup Phrase keeps growing. Remember, the Setup Phrase can be as long as you like, and the more you talk to yourself about the pain, the more likely you are to create descriptions that work.

Even though I have this pain that's the size and shape of a squashed grapefruit in the small of my back...

Even though I have this bright-orange grapefruit-sized pain in the small of my back...

Even though I have this hard, spiky, thorny bright-orange pain the size of a squashed grapefruit in the small of my back...

Even though I have this hard, spiky, thorny bright-orange pain the size of a squashed grapefruit that doesn't make any noise, it's quiet and lethal...

Even though I have this hard, thorny, silent spiky bright red-orange grapefruit pain that shoots flaming lightning bolts that stab like sharp needles through my lower back and up my spine...

This hard, thorny red-orange pain reminds me of when I had a tooth infection and had to go to the dentist, and I felt so helpless and frustrated...

Even though this spiky orange grapefruit pain is interfering with everything in my life so I can't do anything or go anywhere, I can't work, I can't think, it's so frustrating, it makes me so angry, I'm so upset, I feel so helpless, I'm just a wreck, and it's all because of this grapefruit in my back…

11. **When you finish tapping, test your results.** Can you move more easily? Can you stand, sit, bend, walk, or do whatever you couldn't do before? Compare your pain now to the pain you described at the beginning of this exercise. Measure it on the intensity scale. Picture its size, shape, color, and texture. How is it different?

    Now my hard red-orange spiky thorny grapefruit pain is a small square box. It isn't red-orange anymore, it's lime green. It isn't spiky or thorny anymore, it's smooth. It isn't a 10 on the pain scale anymore, it's a 0. It isn't angry and disruptive anymore, it's well behaved and apologetic. It didn't mean to hurt me. I feel safe now. I don't feel helpless. When I bend to the left or right, I can't find any pain at all.

    It was dark brownish yellow and now it's very pale, clear, pastel yellow, almost transparent. It was the size and shape of a golf ball, and now it's smaller than a marble. It hurts a lot less, but I can still feel it when I stand up. I'd say it went from an 8 to a 2 or maybe a 3.

12. **Measure your progress.** If the pain has completely disappeared, congratulations! Enjoy resuming your normal activities. If the pain has improved but has not completely disappeared, start your next round of EFT with *"Even though I still have___"* That's the Setup Phrase to use for whatever pain may be left, for pain

that has moved, and for pain that has changed its shape and size but is still with you.

Even though the pain is still there a little...

Even though I still have some of this pain in a small smooth navy-blue box on the right side of my spine just below my neck...

Even though I still have some of this pain in a soft, round green grape that's stuck in my left shoulder, it's barely a 3, though it's still there, but I can feel it getting softer and dissolving.

The Core Issues of Back Pain

Core issues are the central beliefs or problems that underlie our symptoms. When it comes to back pain, core issues provide the key to rapid relief, if only we can find them and treat them with EFT.

The problem with core issues is that they're not always easy to find. We hide them from ourselves because they're painful. Our subconscious minds don't want us to go there. Our conscious minds are typically unaware of the events or memories lurking beneath the surface or how those events and memories might be causing pain.

In his book *The Divided Mind*, John Sarno, MD, describes tension myositis syndrome, or TMS, as a modern pain-causing epidemic. "In this condition," he writes, "the brain orders a reduction of blood flow to a specific part of the body, resulting in mild oxygen deprivation, which causes pain and other symptoms, depending on what tissues have been oxygen-deprived" (Sarno, 2006).

According to Dr. Sarno, in addition to afflicting millions with back pain, sore necks, painful joints, carpal tunnel syndrome, fibromyalgia, post-polio syndrome, and muscle strains, TMS is the underlying cause of digestive problems such as gastroesophageal reflux, peptic ulcer, hiatal hernia, irritable bowel syndrome, and spastic colitis, as well as tension headache, migraine headache, prostatitis, sexual dysfunction, and tinnitus (ringing in the ears). That's quite a list!

Where does pain come from and why? According to Dr. Sarno, pain serves only one purpose. As noted in the earlier discussion of Dr. Sarno's discoveries, he disagrees with those who believe that pain protects us from further injury or that it has other physiological benefits. Dr. Sarno believes that pain is a reaction to an unconscious emotion and that its sole purpose is to distract the mind from that emotion. He explains:

> Psychosomatic symptoms are created to assist the repression of rage and other unacceptable feelings. Although it is not entirely clear why these unconscious feelings strive to become conscious, it is abundantly clear why the brain resists the attempt. Some of those feelings are believed to be too dangerous or embarrassing or otherwise unacceptable to be brought into the light of day, while others are simply too painful to be experienced consciously. (Sarno, 2006)

To eliminate their pain, Dr. Sarno instructs his patients and readers to recognize pain as a symptom of anger and other negative emotions. He tells them to resume their normal lives instead of lying in bed or restricting their activities. He says that simply understanding the mind-body connection and realizing that their backs hurt because they are angry is enough to cure most patients.

The four sources of rage that Dr. Sarno instructs his patients to watch for are:

1. Harmful emotions, such as anger, hurt, and sadness, that can be traced back to childhood;

2. Anger stemming from self-imposed pressures to be perfect and good;

3. Anger generated by the pressures of life; and

4. Miscellaneous emotions like guilt, shame, insecurity, fear, and vulnerability, which also feed the anger reservoir.

His compelling theory leads straight to EFT, which can effectively and rapidly neutralize harmful emotions, and to our search for the core issues underlying your back pain.

Core Issue Questions

To address your back pain, you could simply say while you tap, "Even though my back hurts, I fully and completely accept myself." If you want to address the pain so it goes away and never comes back, however, it's time to start delving beneath the surface by asking yourself the right questions to lead you to those hidden core issues.

Questions that EFT practitioners routinely ask to start the search for core issues include:

- When did the pain begin?

- What were you doing?
- What was going on in your life?
- Who was with you?
- What happened in your relationship?
- What was going on at work?

Sometimes the answers are obvious. Sometimes they're not. If you can't think of any obvious connections right away, let your mind relax and drift while you think, "If only___." All of us have "if only" moments. They're sad and filled with remorse or regret. "If only I had married Jane…," "If only I hadn't moved to Los Angeles…," "If only I'd stayed in school…"

"If I could do it all over…" is a similar statement. What would you do over? What person or event would you skip if you could live your life again?

The following are further questions and fill-in-the-blank statements that can help you uncover core issues. Again, tap while you ask yourself these questions and fill in the blanks in the statements. Tapping will help relax you, lift any pressure that might be associated with identifying core issues, and avoid unconscious barriers to their discovery.

- What does this back pain remind me of?
- When was the first time I felt this same pain?
- If there is a deeper emotion underlying this pain, what might it be?
- If this back pain were a book or a movie, what would its title be?

- If it were a Broadway play, what would its plot be?

- If I set this back pain to music, what would it be and why—a country song, hard rock, a symphony, a melancholy Argentine tango, a John Philip Sousa march?

- Who or what is the pain in my back? If I could live my life over again, what person or event would I prefer to skip?

- When I relax and let my mind drift, I realize that this pain might have something to do with_____.

- When I think about the pain in my back, I realize _____.

- The worst mistake I ever made was to _____.

- I have this big red ball of rage in my back, and it's all because _____.

The questions may not be necessary if you intuitively know what the core issue is. Some core issues are more difficult to discover, however. In that case, the questions and fill-in-the-blank statements can aid your search.

If you find yourself unable to come up with any answers, you can use EFT to ask your subconscious mind for assistance by tapping while you say:

Even though I can't think of anything right now, I'll let my clever subconscious mind answer these questions with answers that help.

Even though I have no idea where this pain came from or what words to use to find the cause, I choose to effortlessly and effectively allow my brilliant subcon-

scious mind to uncover the core issue and bring the most effective thoughts, ideas, and words to my conscious mind for best results.

Even though my mind is a blank, my brilliant subconscious mind knows what to do to help this technique work.

Sometimes mentioning specific emotions will help trigger a memory. Try tapping while you say:

Even though I might have anger, sadness, guilt, sorrow, hurt, frustration, or other emotions that I can't identify, and they're here under the surface, I love and accept myself, I bless and forgive myself, and even though those feelings are hidden for now, I choose to welcome them as they emerge, knowing that it's safe to invite them into my conscious mind because with the help of EFT tapping, I can be safe in every way, no matter what.

Even though I may have anger in my back, I deeply and completely accept myself.

Even though I can't come up with specific emotions or past events, the truth is that when I think about betrayal, I clearly remember _____.

...when I think about feeling lost and helpless...

...when I think about feeling overwhelmed and confused...

...when I think about that crushing blow of disappointment, as though the floor had fallen out from under me, I remember how my peripheral vision closed in, as though I was in a dark tunnel, and my heart stopped...

You can turn any problem statement into an EFT Setup Statement. For example:

Even though my lower back hurts and it's probably because I'm so worried about money, I choose to replace thoughts of lack with thoughts of abundance. Now my mantra is "All my needs are taken care of."

Even though my middle back hurts, and I just want the world to get off my back, I would like to let go of all the guilt in my back and dwell on the thought that I have released the past and move forward with love in my heart.

Even though my upper back hurts just the way my heart hurts because no one loves me the way I want to be loved, I choose to affirm that life supports and loves me and I love and approve of myself.

If you're still unable to come up with an event, memory, or connection, simply make something up. Engaging the imagination can actually reveal subconscious content. In this way, a made-up example may work even better than an actual event or memory.

As soon as you have something, real or imaginary, that's connected in any way to your pain, create a short or long Setup Statement around it and begin tapping.

EFT can enhance any type of treatment or therapy, which is why so many chiropractors, physical therapists, massage therapists, physicians, personal trainers, nurses, and other health care practitioners incorporate tapping into their professional work. In the following account, Roseanna Ellis, a licensed massage practitioner and physical therapist assistant who uses EFT with chronic pain clients, details two of her cases.

Core Issues Release Severe Back Pain

by Roseanna Ellis

On a Friday night in the summer of 2006, I received a call from a woman begging me to come to her home because she had severe back pain. She said, "I threw my back out and I won't be able to see my doctor until Monday. Please come now."

When I arrived, Mary could barely walk. I treated her in the living room because she was unable to climb the stairs.

I tried all the therapy tricks I knew for about half an hour, to no avail. Then I asked her, "What was happening when you first threw your back out?"

She said, "I was watching my daughter try on her wedding dress." Then she talked about the stress of the wedding and how everything was going wrong. We tapped for the stress, for everything going wrong, and for "I can't take it, I can't rely on anyone."

The pain decreased from a 10 to a 4. She was able to get on and off my treatment table with only slight discomfort, but she was very restricted in range of motion.

I asked her, "Why would your body be afraid to move?"

She answered, "I am a control freak and the wedding planner is not doing things my way and it is freaking me out."

We tapped for:

Even though I am a control freak, I choose to believe that others can also be awesome at what they do. Even though I am a control freak, I choose to give this wedding planner an opportunity to help me. Even though this control freak attitude is causing this immense pain and robbing me of the joy of my daughter's wedding dreams, I choose to get over this nasty habit.

This helped her a lot. She was able to move her body in every direction with a pain level that had fallen to 1. I asked her what was keeping the pain at a 1. She answered, "It is very hard for me to give up control."

We tapped for:

Even though I am making this wedding all about me and not my daughter, I deeply love myself and my daughter.

That did the trick. She sat up with a shocked look on her face and said, "You're right, it is more about me than my daughter." With that, she exclaimed that the pain was a 0, jumped off the table, and gave me a great big hug.

I went over the next morning to give her a good stretch. She was still completely free of pain.

In another case, a 50-year-old man came to see me complaining of intense low back pain that measured a 10 on the 0-to-10 scale. He had very limited range of motion and could not bend over or twist without being in agony.

He was afraid that he would not be able to heal and would have to give up his golf, which he loved so much. He also feared getting old and becoming helpless.

We performed EFT for the issues of being bent over, being afraid of getting old, being afraid to move because of pain, and fearing that he would have to give up golf, his favorite sport.

Within about 15 minutes, his range of motion had improved and his pain decreased to 7. Then he began to speak about his stress at work. We tapped for his stress until his intensity fell to a 0 for stress. His pain fell to 0 and he began to move more easily. We tapped before every motion he performed until all motion was normal and he could twist and bend without pain. In fact, he was able to bend enough to touch the floor. Needless to say, he was very pleased with his session.

❊ ❊ ❊

Aches and pains can be connected to all types of past events, and often you won't realize until you start tapping what memories might be involved. In many cases, the calendar plays a role, subconsciously reminding us of unhappy past events. In this next account, certified EFT practitioner Nancy Privett worked with a woman whose severe shoulder pain turned out to be connected to a painful anniversary.

Shoulder Pain and a Painful Anniversary

by Nancy Privett

Marie came to see me to use EFT for her sore left shoulder and upper arm. This area had been hurting for a few days. The muscles all around the shoulder were sore, as well as the ones going up into her neck and down into her upper arm. She had limited mobility and could not reach behind her to fasten her bra.

I asked Marie what had been going on around the time when she noticed the sore muscles. The only thing that came to her mind was that a few days previously she had been to New York City to see a show with friends and had been holding her purse tightly against her left side with her arm. The next day, she woke up with the soreness.

I noticed that when Marie mentioned her problem she said, "I feel like my mother, all crippled up and can't move." When I asked about that, she said that her mother, who had died 8 years previously and who had lived with Marie and her family for the last several years of her life, had a lot of physical problems, including arthritis in her shoulders.

Several times while talking about her shoulder, Marie repeated the phrase about feeling like her mother, which was a clue that the physical symptoms might be connected emotionally with something to do with her relationship with her mother. However, we began tapping on the physical limitations and pain. Right away, Marie felt a difference. She went from a discomfort level of 8 on the 0-to-10 scale to about a 5. Some phrases we used were:

> *Even though I have this soreness in my shoulder…*
>
> *Even though I can't move my arm the way I want to…*
>
> *Even though I have this pain in my upper arm…*
>
> *Even though it hurts to raise my arm…*
>
> *Even though I can't reach behind my back…*
>
> *Even though this pain goes up into my neck…*
>
> *Even though it hurts more now in my neck than in my shoulder…*

The discomfort was staying at a 5, so I decided to use an EFT approach based on neuro-linguistic programming (NLP). I have had good results with this technique before.

I asked Marie to focus on the discomfort and answer the following as quickly as possible: What color is the discomfort? Is it bigger or smaller than your hand? Is it transparent or solid? Is it moving or still? And, most important: If it were associated with a feeling, what would that be?

To Marie's surprise, the answer to the last question was "sadness." So we tapped on that:

> *Even though I have this sadness in my shoulder…*

Before we had completed the round of tapping, she said, "Oh! Of course!" She then told me that the eighth anniversary of her mother's death was in 3 days, and she was going to be away on a business trip on that day. She began crying, saying that she didn't realize how important it was to be home on that day. (Her mother had died suddenly and unexpectedly at home, in Marie's arms.) We then tapped on:

Even though I am very sad that I won't be home on the anniversary of Mom's death...

When that round ended, Marie said that she had always felt bad about the event of her mother's death because, even though her mother had died in her arms, Marie felt she hadn't said the right things to her as she was passing in order to comfort her. We tapped on:

Even though I feel guilty and bad that I didn't give Mom the comfort she needed as she was dying in my arms...

Even though I didn't say the right thing to her as she died in my arms...

Even though I should have known the right thing to say to comfort Mom as she was dying in my arms...

Notice the reference to the fact that Marie's mother died in Marie's arms, and it was her shoulder and upper arm that were now hurting.

I then suggested to Marie that it really was a lovely and comforting thing in itself that her mother died in her daughter's arms. I said, "Just think, when you die, wouldn't it be nice to be held in the arms of one of your children when it happened?" She said she hadn't thought of that, but it was true.

The session was ending and Marie's shoulder discomfort was still a 5 on the 0-to-10 scale, but she said that "everything feels different." I had an intuitive feeling that after sleeping, her balance would be restored in the morning.

The next morning, she called to say that she felt great and that her shoulder, arm, and neck pain was completely gone. She also felt lighter about her mother's death and didn't feel the sadness that she wouldn't be home for the anniversary. EFT resolved both the physical symptoms and the underlying emotional cause.

※ ※ ※

Bypassing Core Issues

For the record, it is possible to treat back pain with simple Setup Statements that acknowledge core issues without specifically addressing them. For example:

Even though I don't know where this pain came from, it doesn't matter how it started because my body is already, at a deep level, repairing itself, fixing my energy flow, and correcting whatever underlying causes contribute to the pain.

Even though there may be underlying emotional causes for this pain in my back, and my conscious mind doesn't know what they are, it doesn't matter because my subconscious mind is already removing the emotional charge that connects me to events and memories that helped trigger this pain.

Even though I've been trying without success to find the core issues that created this pain in my back, I fully and completely accept myself, and I realize that I may never know what the causes are, and that's okay because my mind and body are already removing the emotional causes, performing subconscious surgery, releasing energy blocks and the pain that they cause.

Even though I feel disappointed and frustrated because I can't figure out where this pain in my back came from or why it had to be there, it truly doesn't matter because I choose to let go of this pain and release it safely and effectively, just by balancing my body's energy.

Even though my conscious mind isn't able to make sense of this pain in my back, I fully and completely accept myself, I love and forgive myself and my back, and I rejoice that my body knows exactly what to do to release this pain and let it go.

Sneaking up on the Core Issue

Sometimes the emotional reason for back pain is an issue so overwhelming that it seems beyond help. It's the "Big One" that we don't want to touch. It may be a major form of guilt we don't want to face or a trauma we don't want to revisit. Whatever it is, we "don't want to go there" and we may even avoid mentioning it to our therapist for fear the therapist will try to drag us through it.

We may have learned to dull the emotional pain associated with it or resolutely refuse to acknowledge it. Regardless, it is still there, under the surface, influencing our thoughts, responses, and everyday lives. Anticipating how upsetting it will be to confront this issue, we would rather endure a less than optimally functional life.

Everything will get better, we hope, if we just address life's minor irritations and leave the "Big One" alone.

Unfortunately, as long as that core issue goes unaddressed, it will continue to constrict your life and, if it is a factor in your back pain, you are unlikely to achieve lasting relief.

Fortunately, EFT has a method for approaching the overwhelming issue in a gentle, nonconfrontive way. You might say you tiptoe up to the issue and circle around it. The method enables clearing the emotional upset of the issue with minimal pain. It begins with a general approach.

Simply say, "*The Big One,* and then rank your 0-to-10 intensity regarding the mere mention of the issue. Rank your pain and other physical symptoms, such as a pounding heart, sweating, constricted throat, and so on. Then use EFT in a general way to help take the edge off:

> *Even though I have discomfort about this issue…*
> *Even though this thing seems too big for me…*
> *Even though just thinking about it bothers me…*
> *Even though my heart is pounding…*
> *Even though (other physical symptoms)…*

For now, you ignore the details of the issue because the main purpose here is to minimize the pain associated with it. You are purposely sneaking up on the problem with gentleness as your goal. Do several rounds of EFT in this more general way until you experience signs of relaxation. A big sigh is a telltale clue.

Next, say again, *"The Big One,"* and re-rank your 0-to-10 intensity on this statement. Chances are your emotional response will be lower and your physical symptoms will likely be down as well. Keep repeating this procedure until you sense that you are ready, comfortable enough, to move on.

Then ask yourself, "Is there any part of this issue that I can talk about comfortably?"

Proceeding in this gentle way often opens the door, making it possible for you to acknowledge or describe at least part of the issue. From there, it is simply a matter of getting more and more detailed. Take some of the edge off, get more detailed. Then take even more of the edge off, and get even more detailed.

You may experience some emotional discomfort in the process. After all, this *is* the "Big One." For most people, however, the discomfort is far less than they feared. Keep in mind, too, that this is probably the last time you will have any such discomfort (if you have any at all). You are clearing the emotional upset you've been carrying regarding this issue. When you have tapped your distress level down to 0, the previously overwhelming issue will have lost its power and will no longer negatively influence your life.

The Tearless Trauma Technique

The Movie and Tell the Story Techniques (see chapter 2) are commonly used in EFT for uncovering core issues. In the case of issues that are emotionally overwhelming, as described in the previous section, these techniques, though gentle, may still be too intense, frightening, or uncomfortable when applied to such cases. If the memory of a traumatic past event is simply too painful to think about, the Tearless Trauma Technique, like the Sneaking Up approach, is a good tool to know how to use.

It is important to remember that, in EFT, you don't have to feel worse in order to feel better. Energy psychology methods such as EFT do not require that you relive a trauma in order to clear the emotional upset associated with it.

The term "tearless" does not mean, however, that no one ever sheds tears or experiences discomfort while using this technique. Tears are often a form of release and people often cry when they experience letting go of a core issue with which they have been burdened their whole lives. The name of the technique refers to the gentle way this is accomplished. In fact, the Tearless Trauma Technique is categorized as one of EFT's "gentle techniques." Please consider it as a method for eliminating distress with a minimum of discomfort.

The technique can be used in any case that involves trauma and is equally applicable to individuals and groups. It has proven especially effective for war veterans, rape victims, and torture victims, but anyone who fears the emotional intensity experienced when speaking or even thinking about a traumatic incident from the past will find the Tearless Trauma approach reassuringly gentle. Though you can use the Tearless Trauma Technique on your own, if your memories entail highly traumatic abuse or violence, you might want to seek the help of a certified EFT practitioner in clearing them. Though the gentle techniques are just that, you may benefit from expert support as you tap your way through them.

While most EFT work involves thinking about details of specific memories and then tapping to neutralize their emotional charge, in the Tearless Trauma Technique you don't focus on the memory. You simply think about the traumatic event from a distance, in the most general way, while tapping.

Here are the step-by-step instructions for the Tearless Trauma Technique.

1. **Select a specific traumatic incident from your past.** Choose something that is at least 3 years old, to minimize any complications from the dynamics of a current event. An example might be "the time my father punched me when I was 12." In contrast, "my father abused me" would be too broad because, chances are, the abuse took place over many incidents. Throughout this exercise, remind yourself to stay on your original issue because it's easy to shift to other issues as you tap.

2. *Guess* **what your emotional intensity would be** (on the 0-to-10 scale) if you were to vividly imagine the incident. Do not actually imagine it (although many people close their eyes and do this anyway). This guess is usually a surprisingly accurate estimate of the emotional intensity of the memory, and it serves to minimize emotional pain because you don't have to replay the painful memory in order to rate its intensity. Write down your guess.

3. **Develop a phrase to use for the EFT process,** such as "this father-punch emotion," and then proceed with a round of tapping.

4. **After this round of tapping, take another guess** as to what your emotional intensity about the subject is now and write it down. It is usually a significantly lower number.

5. **If your emotional intensity is still strong,** perform more rounds of EFT using the same phrase. Three or four rounds brings nearly everybody's estimate down into the 0–3 range.

6. **Perform another round of tapping** once your ratings are down to acceptably low guesses. After this round, try to imagine the incident. Note that this is the first time you are doing so (prior to this you were only guessing at the emotional intensity you would experience were you to imagine the incident). Once again, rate the emotional intensity of the incident. Most people go to 0, but if you do not, address the remaining aspects of the incident with the Movie Technique or Tell the Story Technique (see Chapter 2).

Energy therapies are impressive in their ability to help you process negative emotions. This is particularly clear when using the Tearless Trauma Technique and the other methods described in this chapter to explore sensitive emotional issues contributing to your back pain, a process that might otherwise seem frightening and overwhelming. With EFT, you can delve into previously scary events confident that you have the tools to handle the exploration and approach it as gently as needed.

Resources

Core Issues and How to Find Them:
CoreIssues.EFTUniverse.com

Movie Technique:
MovieTechnique.EFTUniverse.com

Practitioners: Practitioners.EFTUniverse.com

Tapping Circles: TappingCircles.EFTUniverse.com

Tearless Trauma: TearlessTrauma.EFTUniverse.com

Tell the Story Technique:
TelltheStory.EFTUniverse.com

6

Choices, Solutions, and Tapping Tips

In this chapter, we explore a major EFT innovation, the Choices Method, as well as other helpful tapping tips, including what to do when EFT is not producing the results you hoped for in tapping away your back pain.

To review, Clinical EFT focuses on problems. It starts with statements such as "Even though I have this pain in my back..." or "Even though my shoulder is in agony..." and ends with the phrase "I deeply and completely accept myself." The treatment then proceeds with the repetition of a "problem" Reminder Phrase such as the phrase "This pain." There's no doubt that by using this type of Setup Statement, you can tap a problem out.

An EFT innovator, Patricia Carrington, PhD, modified this basic formula, and showed that you can also tap in a *solution*. She did this by adding "I choose" to the last portion of the Setup Statement, making it possible to define or describe a specific desired outcome by inserting an affirmation or positive statement after the words "I choose."

Dr. Carrington, associate clinical professor at the UMDNJ–Robert Wood Johnson Medical School in New Jersey, was one of the first clinical psychologists to incorporate EFT into her professional practice. She not only became a leading EFT practitioner, she also made an important contribution to EFT methodology. Here she describes the technique she developed, which is now widely used in EFT.

The Choices Method
by Patricia Carrington, PhD

When I was using EFT with my own clients in psychotherapy, I soon discovered that I could get even better results if I allowed them to insert their own positive affirmations into the EFT statement. This way the Setup Phrase became perfectly suited to the problems they were addressing.

For example, if a person's hand was throbbing, I would suggest an EFT statement such as, "Even though my hand is throbbing, I choose to have my hand be comfortable and pain free." This immediately makes perfect sense to the injured person; it expresses precisely what they want to bring about—the cessation of pain and the healing of their hand.

It was through experimenting with my own clients that the EFT Choices Method was born. In it, the person applying the method identifies the outcome that they would truly like to have for the problem at hand, and then puts this desired outcome into a phrase that they use at the end of the Setup phrase. Instead of "I deeply and completely accept myself," this phrase commences with the words "I choose."

It's important to note that "I choose" is not used in the format of a traditional affirmation. The latter is a statement that is intentionally contrary to fact, as, for example, when a person living in a dingy basement apartment says, "I live in a beautiful sunny home." This statement is intentionally contrary to fact. According to the rules of traditional affirmations, it will result in subconscious programming that attracts the "beautiful sunny" home of the person's dreams. All too often, however, traditional affirmations result in doubt and skepticism on the part of those who repeat them, particularly if the affirmation is in too sharp a contrast to their current state of affairs.

When people tell themselves that they live in a beautiful sunny home when, in fact, that is obviously not true, the traditional affirmation is apt to create what EFT refers to as a "tail-ender." A little doubting self-statement in the back of our minds says, "Oh, yeah? I know that's absurd!" or "I'll *never* have that!" or "I feel like a fool for saying this."

Such self-doubts are stilled, however, when you place the words "I choose" at the beginning of your affirmation statement. For example, if the person just described were to say, "Even though I live in a dingy basement apartment, I choose to live in a lovely sunny home," the statement would be immediately believable because anyone has the right to make a "choice" and this doesn't contradict the situation the person is in.

This method of injecting choices into EFT soon developed into a definite protocol which I found to be extremely effective, not only for my own clients and workshop participants, but for many others as well. I then formalized the Choices Method and began training other people to use it. It was almost immediately greeted with enthusiasm in the EFT community, and today many thousands of people are using EFT Choices statements. In particular, psychotherapists, counselors, and personal performance coaches are using the Choices Method because it so precisely targets their clients' problems.

❈ ❈ ❈

Dr. Carrington's six rules for phrasing Choices statements are sensible and effective:

1. Be specific.

2. Create *pulling* Choices.

3. Go for the best possible outcome.

4. State your Choices in the positive.

5. Make Choices that apply to you.

Make Choices that are easy to pronounce.

"Pulling Choices" means using words that draw you in and make you feel involved. They are the opposite of dull and boring statements. Dr. Carrington offers the example, *"I choose to express myself in a way that gets my points across to Susan,"* which is a perfectly accurate statement as far as it goes. But, she says, an even more appealing version might be, *"I choose to find a creative way to get my points across to Susan."* As she explains, the word "creative" gives the statement some excitement and suspense. You wonder what would be a creative way to get your points across. "Curiosity is a powerful motivator," says Dr. Carrington. "Surprise" is another word that can draw us in, so another effective statement could be, *"I choose to surprise myself by finding easy and enjoyable ways to get my points across to Susan."* "Easy" and "enjoyable" are pulling words, too, and they help make this a compelling statement.

Here's an example of a Setup Statement that falls short of the six recommendations:

> *Even though my back hurts, I choose to have it not hurt.*

Following Dr. Carrington's suggestions, we can add specific details about the pain, insert some interesting or compelling ideas, describe what we'd rather have, replace negative words (no, not, can't, won't, etc.) with positive words, and create a personally rewarding Choices Statement. For example:

> *Even though I have this sharp, red, throbbing, angry, hard, pyramid-shaped pain stabbing the small of my back just to the left of my spine, I choose to be delighted by how easy it is to enjoy a relaxed, pain-free game of golf tomorrow, with full range of motion, perfect coordination, and my best score yet.*

> *Even though my back has me crying in pain, and I can't believe that this tapping business is going to make any difference at all, I choose to have this whole situation work to my advantage. I choose to have fun doing*

*these EFT exercises in the most ingenious way, with the
enthusiastic cooperation of my brilliant subconscious
mind, so that the whole process is easy, comfortable, and
effortless, and my back feels completely well.*

While tapping on the EFT acupoints, try alternating
between "problem" and "solution" Reminder Phrases.
For example, in the first round of tapping, use "problem"
reminders:

Top of Head: *stabbing pain*

Inside Eyebrow: *so frustrating*

Side of Eye: *terrible pain*

Under Eye: *can't move*

and so on, through all the tapping points.

Or use the same complete "problem" sentence on all
of the acupoints, such as:

Top of Head: *I'm upset because my back is in agony.*

Inside Eyebrow: *I'm upset because my back is in agony.*

Side of Eye: *I'm upset because my back is in agony.*

and so on, through all the tapping points.

Then, in the second round of tapping, use only positive "solution" phrases, such as:

Top of Head: *better already*

Inside Eyebrow: *pain-free*

Side of Eye: *complete range of motion*

Under Eye: *everything's easy*

and so on, through all the tapping points.

— clearing garbage —

(removing)

Or use the same complete "solution" sentence on all of the acupoints, such as:

Top of Head: *I choose to feel completely well in every way.*

Inside Eyebrow: *I choose to feel completely well in every way.*

Side of Eye: *I choose to feel completely well in every way.*

and so on, through all the tapping points.

In the third and final round of tapping, alternate between "problem" and "solution" phrases, such as:

Top of Head: *stabbing pain*

Inside Eyebrow: *I feel wonderful*

Side of Eye: *sharp spasms*

Under Eye: *full range of motion*

Under Nose: *so frustrating*

and so on, through all the tapping points, always ending on a "solution" phrase.

Or alternate between the two complete sentences used previously:

Top of Head: *I'm upset because my back is in agony.*

Inside Eyebrow: *I choose to feel completely well in every way.*

Side of Eye: *I'm upset because my back is in agony.*

Under Eye: *I choose to feel completely well in every way.*

and so on, through all the tapping points.

To be sure your final phrase is positive (you should always end on a positive note), finish by tapping on the Inside Eyebrow point while saying a positive Reminder Phrase.

Some practitioners start with problem Reminder Phrases in the first round of tapping, alternate between problem and solution Reminder Phrases in the second, and devote the third round entirely to solution statements.

Some begin with the basic EFT Setup Statement (*"Even though _____, I fully and completely accept myself,"* or something similar) for their first two Setup Statements and switch to Choices phrasing for the third Setup Statement.

Some use only one Setup Statement and incorporate everything in it before they start tapping the acupoints. Like EFT itself, the Choices Method is flexible, and there is no single "right" way to use it.

The Choices Method is brilliant because it helps people figure out not only what they don't want but also what they do want, it installs affirmations and positive statements, and it helps speed results.

Try it for yourself. Experience is the best teacher. As you experiment with EFT, you will develop your own approach. In the meantime, tap while you read reports about EFT sessions that worked. This simple practice will help you incorporate many different approaches into your EFT repertoire.

When EFT Doesn't Work

EFT can work in the most extreme conditions, when many factors could be expected to interfere with its success, so there are no hard-and-fast rules about when it will work and when it won't. From time to time, however, conditions do interfere. The following are common problems that are easily corrected. If you find that EFT isn't working—you experience no change and the situation seems stuck—try these remedies.

1. There may be a problem with energy in the room.

Try going outside or into another room. There are many possible sources of energy interferences in a room, including electromagnetic fields (EMFs) from electronics, microwaves, or fluorescent lighting, to name a few of the many sources of EMF bombardment in which we live. An easy way to help clear your mind and body is to go outdoors and stand for several minutes with your bare feet on bare ground, grass, sand, concrete, or rocks. The earth supplies a constant supply of free electrons, which are anti-inflammatory and help rebalance energy disturbed by EMF exposure or other energetic interference. Wearing shoes, being indoors, and riding in cars insulates us from those free electrons.

Our modern lifestyles also deprive us of full-spectrum natural light, which our endocrine systems need in order to function well. To remedy that problem, spend as much time as possible outdoors, on a screened porch, or near an open window or doorway—without wearing sunglasses, reading glasses, or contact lenses, all of which prevent the transmission of full-spectrum light. A shady location is fine as long as your eyes have access to natural light.

In addition, being outdoors (assuming the air quality is reasonable) provides fresh air and oxygen. Take several deep breaths, fully inflating your lungs. Then try your Setup Statement and tapping sequence again.

2. It may be something you ate.

A few years ago, one of our practitioners worked with a woman named Abbie who had suffered from depression since the age of eleven. When I first met her, Abbie was suicidal. Tears came easily and "hopeless" seemed to be her favorite word. EFT tapping helped, but whenever her depression lifted a little, it came right back—and this continued after we found and treated several core issues, relieving her back pain and asthma along the way.

During our sixth partially successful session, she felt better until she ate an apple. Within minutes, she was on the brink of a panic attack, her depression shot back to a 10, she behaved as though she had taken a drug, and she fell asleep for several hours.

We invented a "detective diet" to establish what other foods might be causing her problem. She agreed to eat only organic foods (the apple that put her to sleep was not organically grown), eat one food at a time, and wait 1 hour between foods.

From the moment Louella started this detective diet, her depression began to lift and, within 24 hours, it completely disappeared. She began sleeping normally, went on long hikes with friends, enjoyed dancing again, and vacationed in Spain. She learned to avoid wheat, which was the only organic food that triggered an adverse reaction. As long as she stayed away from wheat and commercially grown fruits and vegetables, she felt terrific.

Abbie's food sensitivities are not unusual. Many holistic physicians routinely recommend that their patients stop eating common allergens, such as wheat and dairy products; in many cases, their health improves right away.

Many people who use EFT notice that when they eat certain foods, they soon feel tired, their memory declines, simple projects seem suddenly complicated, and even the simplest EFT tapping requires exhausting effort. In fact, many forget all about EFT. Responses to food are individual, but many experience this kind of fatigue soon after they eat sweets and other carbohydrates.

3. Try varying the Setup Statement.

Try switching from the Karate Chop point to the Sore Spot for your Setup Statement, or vice versa. Also, your Setup Statement may be too general, too global. Make it more specific. Focus on a single incident or a single upsetting detail in an incident. By alternating between the Sore Spot and Karate Chop point and by focusing on the details of upsetting past events, you'll make rapid progress.

4. You may not know what to tap for.

This is not unusual, especially with beginners. It's hard to know what issue to choose, which detail to select, or how to address an issue once you find it. Your subconscious mind can be your ally here. Try using a Setup Statement that invites the subconscious mind to communicate, such as:

Even though I don't know how to use EFT for this problem, I know that my imagination will come up with an appropriate phrase.

Even though I don't know how to define this problem, the right words will come to me without effort.

Even though I can't think right now, I know that deep within me my clever, intelligent mind understands exactly what I hope to accomplish, and it is organizing my thoughts in the best possible way for a good outcome.

5. You may need to do more repetitions.

Focus and perseverance are key to success in EFT. As long as you experience at least some improvement, you are moving in the right direction. EFT practitioners and students often report that when they felt stuck, going nowhere, but continued to tap and tap and tap, suddenly everything shifted.

6. You may be avoiding unhappy memories.

Some people feel uncomfortable saying negative Setup Phrases. They're afraid that thinking about a problem will make it worse. This fear is actually a wonderful tapping subject. By focusing on their fear of tapping, many EFT novices have jumped straight to core issues with excellent results. Example: *I don't want to tap on my weight problem.*

There's your opportunity! Start tapping on:

Even though I don't want to tap on my weight problem, it makes me uncomfortable, I'd rather not even think about it, I don't want to do this, I don't want to think about _____, and I definitely don't want to remember _____.

Let your mind fill in the blanks. Unhappy memories are what make EFT work. Welcome those unhappy memories and start tapping.

EFT is not designed to be a painful procedure. Just tap and think about an unhappy event from a distance, then move a little closer. If it begins to feel painful, back up and tap until the feeling subsides. Then continue. Thanks to EFT tapping, you won't have to relive the experience. You can observe it from a distance without being emotionally involved. This step-by-step procedure, which we call the Tearless Trauma Technique (see chapter 5), has freed people of all ages from the shackles of painful memories while neutralizing core issues that created their pain and discomfort.

7. Try tapping more often.

Try to tap at least five times a day—and more often when you think of it. Set a tapping goal, such as tapping every hour on the hour or at a certain time of day. Tap while you read this book. Find a tapping buddy, someone who can tap with you in person or on the phone, and tap with that person at every opportunity. Recruit friends or family members to form a tapping group. Tap while you watch TV. Tap while you walk the dog. Tap before every meal, whenever you use the bathroom, and whenever you take a bath or shower. Be ingenious about creating time to tap throughout the day.

8. Look for new perspectives.

Try to find a new way of looking at an old, stuck issue. This book introduces many different ways of describing pain. Approach your problem from new directions. Involve your imagination. Think of the problem as a play or movie and put your favorite actors in the cast. Think of it as a computer game and visualize its special effects. Go back to the Personal Peace Procedure (see chapter 2) and work through a dozen different issues.

9. Watch yourself in a mirror as you tap.

Mirror tapping is an excellent way to discover phrases and statements that make you feel uncomfortable. For example, some people are able to say, "I fully and completely accept and love myself," if they're looking at a wall, but not if they're looking at themselves in a mirror. Once EFT neutralizes negative emotions and you install positive emotions and affirmations in their place, mirror tapping can strengthen those positive results, making them a more powerful part of you.

10. Shout it out!

If the Setup Statement isn't getting through, you may not be saying it loudly enough. In EFT workshops and training, we've even had people shout their Setup Statements. Some people do this in their cars with the radio volume turned up. Others do it in the shower. To involve your entire being in this exercise, use emphatic gestures or jump up and down.

11. Get some vigorous exercise.

There's a definite connection between the lymph system and the body's energy system. When you are sedentary, your lymph fluid doesn't circulate well, so the body's waste removal slows down, and that interferes not only with EFT, but also with your overall health and thought processes. Some exciting EFT results have been achieved immediately after a vigorous physical workout. Try jogging, going for a hike, swimming as fast as you can, bouncing on a rebounder (miniature trampoline), or riding a bike immediately before your next tapping session.

12. Clear your energy.

Donna Eden, author of the best-seller *Energy Medicine* (2005) and coauthor of *The Promise of Energy Psychology* (Feinstein, Eden, and Craig, 2008), among other books, has taught thousands of people how to clear their energy and keep it balanced with tapping and other exercises. See her books or videos for instructions.

Try all of the previous suggestions for what to do to improve your outcomes with EFT and keep track of the results so you'll know which strategies work best for you.

In the following article, EFT instructor Barbara Smith offers more helpful suggestions to try when you are not achieving the success you had hoped for from your tapping.

What to Do When EFT Doesn't Work

by Barbara Smith

Have you ever thought, "I tried that EFT and it didn't work," or "How is it that I am tapping all this time and getting so nowhere?" If you have temporarily faltered in your EFT journey, these tips are for you.

1. The One-Minute Wonder

Sometimes, when we first learn EFT, we are fortunate enough to experience or watch one of those amazing demonstrations that result in profound, and seemingly instant, change. We refer to these as "one-minute wonders." They are so exciting and satisfying. They seem so easy and so effective. No wonder people talk about

EFT as the best thing since sliced bread. This kind of transformative success can build our expectation that every session will be like that. When we try it out at home on our own and the problem does not resolve instantly, we feel disappointed and discouraged. We may wonder if there is something the matter with us. Sometimes we lose heart and give up.

The one-minute wonders that you see in demonstrations do occur outside the training room but not in every tapping session. Trainers who work with groups are usually very experienced and able to employ a range of sophisticated EFT techniques. Good trainers make intuitive judgments about which issue to address, the language to use, and the best technique for the situation. If you are a beginner, you are still learning the basics. Keep tapping until the process becomes second nature.

2. When EFT Hasn't Worked *Yet*

It would be easy to head this item "EFT doesn't work for me." This is what disappointed clients say. But when I reframe it as "EFT hasn't worked *yet*," I shift our focus away from failure and we can hold the "yet" as a positive intention.

The metaphor that guides me here and the one I use most frequently is the image of water dripping on a stone. It might take a while to see the effect, but every time EFT "doesn't work," we learn another lesson about ourselves and about what works and what doesn't work for each situation.

3. Do EFT for EFT

When someone tells me that he or she forgot to use EFT at home, or decided not to use it, we might discuss the reasons, and the client may promise to "try harder." At that point, I suggest that tapping now would be useful, and that we will do EFT for EFT.

> *Even though this tapping stuff isn't working, I fully and completely accept myself.*
>
> *Even though I forget to do EFT when it would be really useful...*
>
> *Even though I have messed it up...*
>
> *Even though I give up on EFT before I'm fully over the problem...*

When we have lowered our discomfort, frustration, or anxiety about the EFT not working, we will be free to address the next layer of presenting issues. We may even find some specific events involving our own beliefs about success, and we would tap for those. This meta-level of tapping can be very useful.

4. The "Felt" Experience

One of the ways we know that EFT is really working for us is through "felt" experience. Most adults do not notice the changes in skin temperature, the constant shifts of muscle tension, and the tightness or lack of muscle tone at any moment. When the EFT seems not to be working, you have probably forgotten to notice what is happening in your body.

It is very useful to stop and notice exactly what has changed. Has the tension gone out of your chest, are your shoulders tense or relaxed, or has the mental picture changed? Does your body feel lighter, your breath easier? Has the thought changed? Teach yourself to notice these changes using all of your senses. Later, you can refer back to the specific experience to find what you might be overlooking or to recapture the feeling of success that you previously discovered.

5. EFT Will Never Work for Me

There are some situations where beginners can give up or feel hopeless. There are many reasons that may stop you from reaching instant success. One reason is Psychological Reversal. When we first learn EFT, we begin to work on ourselves using the basic skills. We don't have enough experience and confidence to treat some deeper issues. This is the time to work one-on-one, in person, by phone, or in a group with an experienced practitioner who is familiar with the more sophisticated applications of EFT and who will help you recognize and address core experiences and hidden beliefs that may block you from change.

6. What Words Were You Using?

When people tell me that EFT didn't work, I ask for specific information about the issue, its aspects, and the phrases the client was saying. This is the way to get specific about what happened or where the protocol might be improved. Write down the issue, the Reminder Phrase you are using, and the intensity level of your distress in relation to this issue. This is especially important if you are working on your own. Note every change in aspect and intensity after each round. In this way, you will be able to look back and remind yourself of your progress and previous successes. If you are helping someone else with EFT, this record will ensure you can quickly identify any issues that may have been overlooked.

7. Too Much Too Fast?

Because EFT is not working at home does not mean that EFT will not work. It just means it has not worked *yet*. Sometimes the reason is that we have tried to address one of our truly big issues, one whose distress level is overwhelming. Try some practice sessions on less intense issues, or choose a less arousing aspect of your problem before going back to the *big one*.

8. The EFT Skeptics Society

Most of us have had years of experience of using the thinking-talking-trying harder process of therapeutic change and, in the beginning with EFT, we may find ourselves drifting back to a talk model because we find it very difficult to believe that something as strange as EFT will really work.

Those of us who are health professionals know that many of our colleagues are still skeptical about EFT. I remember that it took me some time before I routinely used EFT on myself. I chose a few colleagues with whom to share what I was learning and gradually became more confident about presenting EFT to others.

Now I use it on everything and cannot imagine how I ever lived without EFT.

Find a friend, colleague, or professional who knows and uses EFT. If you don't know any EFT person near you, arrange some telephone coaching, subscribe to an EFT newsletter, and read accounts from others about their success with EFT. Keep up-to-date with innovations through Internet newsletters. Support may be the very thing that makes the difference.

Once you have achieved a high rate of success with EFT in your own life, other people's skepticism does not matter. You can change your response to others with a little tapping: *Even though I really hate the way she rolls her eyes when I mention EFT...*

9. Testing, Testing, Testing

Are you testing at home? What are you testing?

In my practice, this is the thing that new clients find the most difficult to do consistently at home. Is it possible that you wandered off target?

Before you decide that EFT is not working for you, write down your distress level and the problem's aspects for every round. Some issues take several rounds before they clear completely. I suggest to my clients that if they think there is no change, they should be prepared to do up to five rounds at any one level of intensity before they move to a new aspect or topic. If you carefully record your intensity rate and are clear about the aspect you're treating, you will probably find yourself making progress.

10. Back to Basics

The EFT Manual (Church, 2013; Craig & Fowlie, 1995) remains the definitive source of EFT theory and practice. Experienced therapists have been integrating EFT with numerous other psychological and physiological forms of healing, and also creating variations on EFT that we sometimes call EFT's "cousins." If EFT is not working for you, check to be sure in your sessions at home that you are following all of the EFT basics as detailed in this book and in *The EFT Manual* (Church, 2013).

Then, in the words of family therapist Virginia Satir, "Try it on everything and swallow only what fits."

Resources

Choices Method by Patricia Carrington:
Choices.EFTUniverse.com

Core Issues and How to Find Them:
CoreIssues.EFTUniverse.com

Practitioners: Practitioners.EFTUniverse.com

Tapping Circles: TappingCircles.EFTUniverse.com

Tearless Trauma: TearlessTrauma.EFTUniverse.com

When Your Client Feels Worse:
ClientFeelsWorse.EFTUniverse.com

7

EFT in Action
for Back Pain

There are so many ways in which EFT has relieved pain that it is beyond the scope of this book to describe them all. This chapter, however, offers multiple reports from EFT practitioners and instructors to give you an idea of the range of possibilities for relieving your back pain when you start tapping. While you read the accounts, tap your EFT points. This can actually help with your own back pain. If a story resonates with you, try inserting your own situation in the tapping language and see what results you get.

In the first article, EFT Master practitioner Maggie Adkins suggests three approaches to exploring your pain.

Three Methods for Working with Pain
by Maggie Adkins

There are numerous ways to work with pain using EFT. Sometimes pain just shifts while you are working on another issue. That issue could be anything—past trauma, anger, grief, sadness, or myriad other issues. At other times, you may want to do EFT while focused specifically on pain. Here are three ways to work with pain in the body.

1. Focus on the actual pain.

Even though I have this lightning bolt pain in my side...

Even though I have this throbbing headache in the front of my head...

Even though I have this dull ache in my left knee...

2. Focus on how you feel about the pain.

Even though I'm afraid if this pain keeps up, I won't be able to dance anymore...

Even though I'm terrified I'll lose my job if this pain gets worse...

Even though if I were the person I think I am, I would have gotten rid of this pain long ago...

Even though I have these emotions about having this pain...

3. Find an emotion or quality in the pain or part of the body in pain.

Even though I have this resentment in my shoulder...

Even though I have this anger in my lower back—nobody ever supported me and I'm tired of doing it all myself...

Even though I have this shame/grief/sadness (whatever it is) in my back...

These are just a few ideas. Use your genius and your intuition.

✿ ✿ ✿

Now we'll take a look at some of those famous EFT "one-minute wonders." The term refers to the nearly instant results that sometimes occur in EFT, that is, someone does a few rounds of tapping and the back pain or other problem disappears. Sometimes it even happens after just one round. In the following report, Graham Batchelor, who runs a sports injury clinic in the United Kingdom, shares how astonished he was when he tried EFT for the first time with a client and the severe pain from the client's back injury disappeared.

Pain from Severe Lower Back Injury Resolved

by Graham Batchelor

The free introduction manual to EFT whetted my appetite and I ordered all the available material. After it arrived, I became so enthralled that I spent almost all my time over the next 2 weeks engrossed in it. I must confess I neglected my sports injury clinic, but something told me that EFT was the way forward and the more knowledge I could gain, the better my results with treatments would be.

This was proven correct during an appointment with a 45-year-old man who told me that, after a serious injury to his lower back at work, he had been hospitalized for 6 months and confined to a wheelchair for a further 2 years. Physiotherapists had worked with him over this period and eventually got him walking with the aid of crutches, but he was only able to cover about 30 meters (100 feet) at a time. Although he was on powerful analgesics, he still suffered a large amount of pain, and he had been told that little more could be done for him.

When he arrived for our appointment, I could tell from his efforts to walk that his lower back and legs were pain-ridden. His posture was very lopsided, and he was completely exhausted from the effort to get to me. He found it very difficult to get onto the treatment couch but insisted on doing so.

Although I had only just gained a small understanding of EFT, I began talking through the problems he had faced since the injury. It became obvious that he felt exceptionally guilty about his inability to help his wife when cancer struck and she underwent a major operation. He was also concerned that his earning power had dropped to zero. He indicated his quality of life was only a 2 on the "positive" 0-to-10 scale.

I gained his permission to try EFT with him and began with the Karate Chop point. We went through a basic Setup procedure using:

> *Even though I have this serious injury…*
>
> *Even though I could not help my wife in her time of urgent need…*
>
> *Even though I can no longer support my family…*

When we reached the collarbone point, he began sobbing, his breathing became labored, and his lower body began twitching. We stopped and I explained that

I thought he was going through a very strong emotional release. He gradually regained composure and we carried on.

At the end of the second round, he requested that we continue, indicating he felt much better emotionally and his pain was reducing. After the third round, I prepared to help him off the couch. Amazingly, he stood by himself and, using only one crutch, began walking around the treatment room.

I advised him not to be too adventurous and to take things a little easy. With tears of happiness in his eyes, he could not thank me enough. I explained that EFT and he himself were the healers and I was only a channel. Talking through his treatment, he now said he felt his quality of life had gone to a wonderful 9 out of 10 and he could not wait to get home to his wife. I talked to him and his wife 3 days later and neither could believe his recovery.

After running a sports injury clinic using shiatsu, Reiki, and other healing techniques for almost 20 years, I cannot believe how EFT helped this patient. I intend to use it at every opportunity. I look forward to getting much more experience and understanding, but for this first attempt, I truly am amazed.

※ ※ ※

Graham was concerned about his client's welfare when he warned him not to do too much now that he felt better, but often when we let go of the emotional factors that keep us in pain, we can safely resume our normal activities. If, as a result of your back pain, however, it has been a long time since you have engaged in what used to be normal activities for you, please practice common sense in taking up those activities again. Your body will likely need to rebuild its physical strength. Consult your doctor if you have any questions about appropriate activities for you. And remember, EFT is always there for you to use as a first-aid treatment, for example, for easing soreness in muscles suddenly become active after long disuse.

If you would like to work on your back pain with an EFT practitioner, your choice of practitioner need not be limited by geographical location. EFT can be conducted by phone or via Skype or other online modality. Many practitioners work this way so they can help people who might otherwise not have access to an EFT professional. Working via phone or Skype is especially helpful for people with severe back pain, as travel, even locally, may be too difficult. In the following report, EFT practitioner Aileen Nobles details her highly effective phone work with a back pain client.

Eight Months of Chronic Back Pain Disappears

by Aileen Nobles

When I spoke to Joanie on the phone, she was terrified and desperate. She was in so much pain and yet so afraid of having a session that she had previously canceled me twice. The third time she kept her phone appointment. She suffered from chronic pain down the right side of her neck and shoulder, down her back and into her arm and hand. This pain had been going on for 8 months and she told me she had only had a couple of hours' sleep a night for many months. She had not been able to work, was depressed, and was at her wits' end. Her pain level was consistently at a 9 or 10 on a scale of 0 to 10.

When I asked her what happened in her life around 8 months ago, she couldn't remember anything of importance. I explained that our bodies have almost unlimited restorative healing capabilities if there is a free flow of energy in the meridians. Whenever our physical body is feeling less than perfect, it is asking us to look at our emotional body. Something had probably happened around the time this pain started.

Intuitively, I knew that working on the pain alone was not going to produce the change I wanted. The fact that she had canceled me twice and was so afraid led me to believe some kind of emotional trauma was being suppressed. Again I asked her if anything out of the ordinary had happened 8 months ago when this pain started. She couldn't think of anything.

I mentioned that, even though she couldn't think of anything right now, her subconscious and superconscious were both holding the necessary information. I suggested we start tapping and we would see if anything came up.

Even though I can't remember what happened 8 months ago...

Even though part of me may be afraid to remember if anything happened that was very upsetting, I'm still quite wonderful anyway.

We moved to the Gamut point and tapped on:

My subconscious knows if anything happened, and my superconscious is always protecting me.

I would like to believe that I am in safe hands, and it's safe for me to bring any situation connected with my pain into my conscious mind.

Bingo! Joanie blurted out that 8 months ago her mother had died. Yes, that was a painful experience! Joanie's mother had always been a strong support system, helping Joanie to believe in herself. She depended on her mother so much that she had always been afraid that without her mother she wouldn't want to live. Joanie was married to a very sweet and gentle man, and when her mother crossed over, she didn't want him to know that she felt like dying. She didn't want him to feel that her mother meant more to her than his love for her.

She had so much internal pain connected with the loss of her support system — her mother — and guilt over not wanting to hurt her husband that she stuffed it all inside. She chose not to deal with it to the point of blocking it out...but her physical body had other ideas. We tapped on:

My husband loves me so much he does not want me to be in pain and it's okay to talk to him about how much I miss my mother.

I'm safe and loved and he will understand how I feel.

Now that I am safe enough to acknowledge my inner pain, it no longer needs to manifest as outer pain.

Thank you, wonderful physical body, for bringing my attention to emotions that needed to be addressed.

We did a few rounds on releasing the sadness.

I have a lot if pain inside as I miss my mother so much.

Joanie then held the points under her eyes without tapping. *My pain on the inside is manifesting on the outside, I'd like to let it go.* She took three deep breaths. *My pain on the inside no longer needs to manifest on the outside as I allow myself to release it.* She took three more deep breaths, and we began to reframe the loss. Joanie acknowledged that her mother would not want her to be sad and in pain, and being sad wasn't accomplishing anything useful. Her mother would want her to become strong and enjoy her wonderful husband. We continued tapping:

The last thing my mother would want is for me to be in pain.

My mother always wanted me to be happy with my husband.

Joanie's level of pain was now down to 2 out of 10 and was in her neck. We continued tapping:

Even though I have this 2 pain in my neck, I really am terrific anyway.

Even if this pain in my neck is me, I'm still quite wonderful anyway.

I don't need to be a pain in the neck to myself or anyone else, I'm ready to heal and be happy and productive.

She laughed out loud and said the pain was all gone, and she was looking forward to speaking openly with her husband. Joanie no longer had any guilt connected with not loving her husband enough, as she accepted how we love different people differently. Her love for her husband was very special in its own unique way.

We talked about her going back to work and feeling as if she had a purpose. She was so amazed and excited that she was pain free and felt so different from the way she had at the beginning of the phone call. She did start working again with her husband and is still pain free.

Again and again, I see pain and illness lift and disappear even when painkillers are not having any effect. What an incredible tool we have in our own hands.

❀ ❀ ❀

It isn't every day that attorneys relieve their clients of back pain. Notice how attorney Ted Robinson aims EFT at emotional issues to clear up his client's pain. Notice also how the client tries to "explain away" the result. This often happens with astonished newcomers to EFT. They have a hard time believing that fingertip tapping could have such immediate and profound effects.

Attorney Relieves Client's Back Pain

by Ted Robinson

I was with a young woman who was charged with two felonies for forging a prescription for oxycodone, which she said she had to do because of severe back pain after an auto accident. She claimed her insurance ran out and the doctor wouldn't give her any more prescriptions, so she arranged to have some blanks given to her and she forged them to get her pain relievers. She said she had a ruptured disc between L-4 and L-5. Of course, as soon as we left the court, I suggested we give EFT a try.

Her 0-to-10 intensity was a 6 or 7. Then after a simple Setup of "This pain in my back that's a 7," I started the Sequence with "This pain in my back" and repeated it as we went through the points. I was shortly drawn to add other wording like:

Even though I'm carrying my whole family around on my back…

Even though it's not fair…

Even though I have the entire responsibility for our entire family on my shoulders and back…

Within about 90 seconds, I noticed her moving her back to check to see if it still hurt. Her expression was somewhat quizzical and she looked at me and said, "It feels better…much better. But you made me think about all that tapping instead of my back, right?"

I said no, it was just the energy being balanced and the underlying issues being recognized. She was much happier and relieved knowing she had a new way to deal with her pain. She also realized that if she'd had such a method ahead of time, she would never have been arrested or be facing jail time.

❊ ❊ ❊

In the next account, EFT Expert practitioner CJ Puotinen describes another EFT phone session that alleviated back pain. Notice the length of some of the Setup Statements, demonstrating how to include numerous details. Note, too, the application of Dr. Carrington's Choice Method in the statements.

Three-Week Back Pain Relieved in Phone Session
by CJ Puotinen

While confirming registrations for an upcoming workshop, I left a phone message for Holly Anne Shelowitz, a nutrition counselor in Kingston, New York. When Holly called back, she explained that she hadn't replied to my e-mails because she hadn't been able to access her computer for 3 weeks. She had injured her back and had been in bed that whole time. Friends were staying with her in shifts 24 hours a day because she needed help doing everything. Every movement was excruciatingly painful.

"I don't know anything about EFT," she said, "but I was wondering if there is some way I can get started now, before the workshop, in case it would help with the pain."

I asked her to describe the pain, beginning with its size, shape, and location. She said it had at first covered her entire back, but it was now in the small of her back. In response to my questions (is it bigger than a breadbox, is it square or round, what is its three-dimensional shape, is it soft or hard, is it smooth or rough, what color is it, does it make a sound, does it move or pulse?), she described it as the size and shape of a slightly squashed grapefruit, red-orange in color, with a hard spiky, thorny surface, not making any noise, and not moving or pulsing.

We slowly went through the EFT tapping points. She used a phone headset, which freed her hands for tapping, and soon she was tapping along at a good clip, saying,

> *Even though there's a pain in the small of my back that's the size and shape of a slightly squashed hard red-orange grapefruit, and it's covered with thorns and spikes, and it's just stuck there and it won't move except to cause a lot of pain whenever I move, and it has turned me into an invalid, in fact I'm a total mess, I fully and completely accept myself.*

> *Even though this pain is overwhelming and it's kept me flat on my back for three weeks and my back is a mess and my life is a mess, I fully and completely accept myself, I love and forgive myself, I forgive this pain, I forgive my back, and I choose to be pleasantly surprised at how easy it is to relax and let go of this pain and feel better.*

> *Even though this tapping business is very strange, I'm desperate enough to try anything and, who knows, maybe it will unblock some blocked energy and let my meridians flow the way they're supposed to, and maybe I'll feel a little better in a few minutes.*

These statements were interspersed with the EFT point tapping, starting at the top of her head, the third eye at the center of her forehead, inside eyebrow, outside eye, under the eye, under the nose, under the lip, collarbone, under the arm, and several taps across the upper abdomen. My husband's Tibetan acupuncturist suggested that rather than focus on a specific liver point, we tap all over the upper abdomen, from waist to partway up the rib cage and from far right to far left, because several meridians run through that area, and the more places we tap, the more likely we are to hit meridians that will help.

At each tapping point, I had Holly say a different Reminder Phrase: *pain, hurts, red-orange, hard, spiky, thorns, rough, hard, difficult, squashed grapefruit,* and so on.

After a few quick rounds of head-to-torso tapping, Holly sounded more relaxed. I assumed that her pain was diminishing, but I wanted to give her a good foundation for future reference, so instead of asking how she felt, I taught her the hand points, explaining that she might not need them, but it's good to know how to use them, just in case. We completed the finger tapping by tapping the fingertips of the right hand against the nails of the left hand, and vice versa.

After a few rounds that incorporated the hand points, we did the 9 Gamut Procedure. I called it the "brain balancer" and explained that it brings the left and right brains into balance. Holly was happy to learn this simple procedure.

Then I asked Holly how she felt about the pain. Soon she was saying, while tapping on her Karate Chop point:

> *Even though I'm furious with this pain, totally angry and upset, here I am stuck in bed, not able to work, not able to go anywhere, not able to do anything*

by myself, dependent on everyone, it's so frustrating, my body betrayed me, I have no control over my body or anything, it's so upsetting!

Even though I hate all this, I fully and completely accept myself, I love and forgive myself, I forgive myself for hurting my back, I forgive my back for being hurt, I forgive anyone and anything that had anything to do with my being in this condition, and I choose to amaze myself at how easy it is to let go of this hard, thorny, excruciating red-orange spiky pain, to let it go, to release it and everything that has contributed to it in any way, and I choose to be completely well, I choose to let my body heal itself from the inside, I choose to relax and be happy, and that's the truth!

Tap tap tap tap tap with appropriate Reminder Phrases: *angry, frustrated, body betrayed me, upset,* and so on, followed in the next round by positive Reminder Phrases: *let go, release, forgive, love, good back, strong back, happy back.*

Just to be sure we were clearing everything that might be a factor, I started Holly on a new Setup Phrase, saying:

Here I am stuck in bed, I've been here for three weeks, life is passing me by while I stare at the ceiling, I may be here forever, and I find, as I lie here thinking about everything, that this reminds me of _____.

Holly stopped, then realized that I was waiting for her to fill in the blank. "This reminds me of when I had an infected tooth," she said, "and I was lying in the dentist's chair with all that cotton and stuff in my mouth, totally helpless, not in control of anything, not able to move because of a condition I could do nothing to fix. It was the most awful feeling. I was afraid and upset and helpless, and I think feeling helpless is what bothered me the most."

So we tapped on:

Even though I feel helpless, just as helpless as when I was stuck in the dentist's chair, and even though I have to rely on friends for help to do everything because I'm helpless, and even though I can't do anything for myself, can't work, can't walk, can't sit up, can't do anything by myself or for myself, I'm as helpless as a baby, I'm paralyzed, I'm stuck, I'm helpless, nevertheless I fully and completely accept myself, I love myself, I love my back, I forgive myself and my back and everything and everyone for anything and everything, and I choose to be completely well, I choose to release all this and let it go, I choose to say goodbye to the pain.

I know that in some way this pain that has kept me in bed for 3 weeks was my body's attempt to keep me safe, so with gratitude I thank the part of me that controls this pain, I love and bless it, I acknowledge its excellent work, it has done its job very well, and now that it realizes that the useful purpose it served is now complete, it can let go now, right now, and it can know how much I appreciate its good work. It can come back when it's needed and necessary, and for now it can let the pain subside, it can release the pain, it can let go while I thank it for doing such a good job. I choose to be delighted at how easy it is to let the pain go, and the part of me that controls the pain can thoroughly enjoy how easy it is to release this pain now. I thank this pain, I bless this pain, and I release this pain now.

At the end of all this, Holly sighed a deep, deep sigh, a good sign that her energy was shifting. And now when she laughed, it wasn't a nervous pain-filled laugh, it was a relaxed laugh, a laugh with relief and a spark of hope and joy in it.

I asked Holly whether her pain was still the size and shape of a slightly squashed grapefruit.

"No!" she exclaimed. "It's a little cube, like a small box, and it isn't red-orange any more, it's a deep velvet blue, and it isn't rough and spiny anymore, it has a smooth velvet surface. It's almost gone!"

Now we tapped on:

Even though I have this small velvet blue box of pain in the small of my back, I fully and completely love and accept myself. Even though there is still a little box of blue velvet pain in the small of my back, the pain is disappearing, it is going away, my body is healing itself from the inside out, I feel better already, I feel so much better, I really feel completely well.

At the end of two or three rounds of tapping, Holly couldn't find the pain at all. It had disappeared.

"Okay," I said, "let's see if we can find it again. Do you feel like sitting up?"

Holly realized that she probably could, and she did. I asked her to bend to the left, right, forward, and back to see if she could find the pain, and she couldn't. It was gone.

"Feel like standing up?" I asked.

"Oh, gosh," said Holly. "Do you think I should? I mean, do you think I can?"

"Well," I said, "your friend is there to help."

Her friend had, in fact, been rolling his eyes as he watched Holly tap and talk, but now he had something useful to do, so he stood beside her as she took a tentative move toward standing.

"I can't!" she cried and sat back. But it was not pain that interfered this time, it was fear. We tapped on:

Even though I'm afraid to stand, I feel dizzy, I'm afraid I'll fall, I think I'll faint, I'm afraid I'll injure myself all over again and I'll be right back where I started. I'm afraid this won't work. I'm afraid to try. I'm too afraid to think straight. On the other hand, I trust my strong, healthy body, which is healing itself from the inside out. I trust my brilliant mind, which is directing all my nerves and muscles to stand me up straight and keep me there. I love and trust my body and mind and nerves and bones and muscles and everything else. I choose to let go of the fear. I'm going to stand up now.

And she did! Holly was amazed. She kept laughing. "I can't believe it! I'm standing up! It was so easy!" And she couldn't find the pain, even when she leaned to the left, right, forward, and back, and even when she bent her right leg and pulled it toward her, then did the same with her left leg. She felt a little stiff from all that bed rest, but we tapped on the stiffness and she soon felt more limber.

Then she said, sounding shy and tentative, like a little girl, "It's such a beautiful day, it's so lovely outside, I wonder—do you think that maybe—could I maybe—do you think I could, well, could I go for a walk? Outside? By the lake?"

I burst out laughing. "Tap with me," I said.

Even though I've spent the last half hour lying on my back, tapping on my head, and saying all kinds of ridiculous things with someone I've never met in my life, and now I'm asking this total stranger who's 70 miles away for permission to go for a walk...Do I need my head examined?

We zipped through the tapping points, saying:

Going for a walk! I feel terrific! Going outside! Beautiful day! The end! Goodbye!

Holly and her friend took a 20-minute walk by the lake, and she felt completely fine. She immediately resumed her work and her normal activities. Nearly 2 years have passed since Holly's introduction to EFT, and during that entire time she has felt only an occasional minor twinge of pain, especially when she's under stress. Whenever that happens, she taps and the pain disappears.

❀ ❀ ❀

Resources

Choices Method by Patricia Carrington:
Choices.EFTUniverse.com

9 Gamut Procedure: 9Gamut.EFTUniverse.com

Practitioners: Practitioners.EFTUniverse.com

Tapping Circles: TappingCircles.EFTUniverse.com

When Physical Symptoms Resist Healing:
SymptomsResistHealing.EFTUniverse.com

8

EFT as First Aid

Some of my favorite reports are from both newcomers and those experienced in EFT who use tapping as a first-aid treatment. As the accounts in this chapter show, this can be an effective strategy not only for accidents or episodes of back strain or pain that just occurred, but it can benefit old injuries as well. In the first report, the client was a newcomer to EFT who used it on herself. No outside assistance was involved or needed.

Back Pain Subsides After 14 Years

by Evelia A. Sanchez

Fourteen years ago, my friend was hit by a bus and was left with terrible neck and back problems. She was in so much pain that she would go into spasms during which she could move only by hobbling and dragging one leg.

She went to many different doctors and healers but found only temporary relief for her now-crooked back and disabling pain. Her best relief came from a chiropractic treatment, but the results were only temporary and she had to go every 1 to 3 months. She had done this for the past 13 years. It was terribly expensive for a woman on a small pension.

When I realized that EFT could help her, I taught it to her. I instructed her to do the work as often as she could and to let me know what happened. That was a year ago and I am proud to let everyone know that she has not needed a back adjustment in all that time.

For the first month, she tapped every time she was in pain. Her back shifted quickly and the pain shifted dramatically. She could feel tingles go up and down her spine as she worked on it and that's how she knew something was changing.

She continued to go to the chiropractor just to monitor her back with X-rays, but she has not needed to have her back adjusted since starting EFT. She says that, on her last visit, the doctor told her that her back was almost perfectly aligned. He was so happy to report this, and he believes it was his work that helped her.

I begged her to tell him about EFT, but she says he is not open to it and she does not want to offend him. Oh, well. We know the truth and he has documented it for us. Great job, EFT!

✻ ✻ ✻

In the following case, Peggy Lawson used EFT to relieve her dentist's substantial back pain. In the process, she "borrowed benefits" and reduced her own dental pain and discomfort. The phenomenon of Borrowing Benefits (see Chapter 10) is one of the many advantages we receive when we tap on behalf of others, as Peggy did, or tap along with someone working on an issue. Your own circumstances, whatever they are, improve without conscious effort on your part.

How I Fixed My Dentist's Back Pain

by Peggy Lawson

I had an appointment at the dentist the other day. He had already canceled a previous appointment because he had hurt his back.

When I arrived at his office, the dental assistant informed me that he was still in a lot of pain, but he was working because he didn't want to disappoint any more of his patients. When the dentist walked in, I could see the pain in his eyes. It occurred to me that I truly didn't want anyone who was in that much pain working in my mouth.

I asked him if he could think of any emotional reason for the pain in his back and he said, "No, I don't think so. And it's not exactly in my back, it's more in my, ahem, lower left cheek."

When I asked him if he was willing to allow me to show him something that might help him, he recoiled and said, "Will it hurt?" My eyes slid over to the huge syringe with the 4-inch needle that he was preparing to stick in my jaw, and I replied dryly, "Not as much as that's going to hurt me!"

He was desperate and willing to try anything. So I sat up in the chair, and we did four rounds of EFT.

Even though my lower back hurts…

Even though I have this pain in my left cheek…

Finally, I said:

Even though I have a big pain in my ass…

Which, after two rounds, left him chuckling, but more important, pain free. Free to work on me next! This next part is incredible to me.

I don't have any phobias about going to the dentist, but it's not something I look forward to, either. I hate when the needle goes into my jaw, and I really dislike the way the numbness makes my lips feel 10 sizes larger and I can't even tell if I'm drooling or not. The numbness taking its time to wear off is very unpleasant also, and I sometimes bite the inside of my mouth until it does. I had none of that!

I didn't even feel the needle going into my gum, and I never felt any pain or any unpleasant numb feeling. It was as if I hadn't needed an anesthetic at all. It was amazing to me. Apparently, since I had spent several minutes tapping for and with him, I borrowed the benefits of EFT from the dentist! I can't remember when that's ever happened to me before, and I tap on a lot of people!

I highly recommend tapping for your dentist next time it's necessary to go, if he or she will let you, and see if it doesn't help you!

❈ ❈ ❈

In this next report, Dr. Larry Stewart was about to call for an ambulance after his wife pinched a nerve in her back. Thanks to EFT, the ambulance wasn't needed.

EFT Cancels an Ambulance Call

by Dr. Larry Stewart

Two weeks ago, at 8:00 on Saturday morning, I awoke to hear my wife's cries of pain. Shirley had picked up a stack of magazines and, in the process, had pinched a nerve in her back (she's done it before) and was lying on the ground, crying from the pain. I started to call an ambulance, but I decided to see if I could offer some immediate relief from some of the pain. She rated the pain in her back as a solid 10 and the numbness in her toes rated an 8 on the big toe and 10 on the small ones.

We tapped, but no change. We tapped again, and she felt a little relief. After about 15 rounds of tapping, she was down to 1 on the back pain, 0 on the numbness in her big toe, and 2 or 3 on the numbness in her smaller toes. She rested and continued to tap every few hours through the weekend. We finally got her to her physician and chiropractor on Monday.

For the next few days, anytime the pain crept up, she would tap. She continued to tap for the numbness. Ten days later, she was able to walk normally again. Whenever she had pinched a nerve before, it meant days in bed followed by months of pain and numbness. I'm convinced that EFT helped, at least to relieve the neuro-muscular tension that accompanied the injury.

❅ ❅ ❅

Many people who were injured in a car crash or other emergency situation have described how tapping reduced their pain, kept them calm, and helped them cope with whatever happened before and after the accident. When Barbara Cohn totaled her car, the first thing she did was focus on EFT.

EFT and My Car Crash

by Barbara Cohn

Day before yesterday, I was in a really bad car accident in New York City. In fact, my car was totaled. I'd been studying EFT for a few months and had just completed the Level 2 and Level 3 workshops, so, faced with the shock of being in an accident and not really sure what happened, I began tapping. Right away, I was interrupted by helpful bystanders who opened my car door and proceeded to check me out and tell me not to move and that an ambulance and the police were coming. I ached all over, but I could move all my parts and the only blood was from where the seatbelt scraped my neck and where I bit my tongue.

Before I could begin tapping in earnest, the ambulance arrived and the paramedics used the standard things like a collar and back board, even though I knew I didn't need them and said so. Getting me from the car using the back board and the collar really hurt, partly because I am not a skinny woman and partly because the way they did it really hurt my bruises!

As soon as I was in the ambulance and lashed to the board and gurney, I began tapping about my aches and shock and the trauma of the car hitting the metal stanchion of the overhead subway. I knew that the paramedics who were writing up stuff would think I needed psychiatric help if they heard me doing Setups so I said the phrases in my head and physically tapped on the Karate Chop point, and then the crown chakra on the top of my head, the third eye, the face points, the collarbone, the under the arm, and the abdomen rib points. When that didn't seem enough, I tapped on the finger points.

I tapped for my guilt about totaling the car and said I forgive myself even though I still wasn't sure what had happened. I tapped for the driver of the other car, who claimed I hit him, and I forgave him because I didn't know whether he was right or wrong, and at that point it didn't matter. I can't remember all the Setup Statements I used because I tapped on everything I could think of, including my son's reaction to the loss of the car and my daughter's reaction to the fact that she now had no car to use. I even did a mental movie and saw myself hitting the pole and being unable to move out of the way. I wasn't tired, but each round of tapping produced yawns, so I knew something was happening. In the hospital, they put an IV needle in my arm in case it was needed, so imagine, if you will, tapping one-handed because of being lashed to a board, attached to a collar to prevent you from moving your neck, with tape over your forehead to keep you still on the gurney, and with an IV needle in your arm.

At the hospital, it was hurry up and wait because I wasn't logged in right away, so I kept tapping about my bruises, aches and pains, how awful the board was, the pain in my head from being on the board, and the bruise at the Gamut point that was black and swollen but not painful. I tapped for my swollen and bleeding tongue and how it hurt to swallow around the lump in my throat. I even did one 9 Gamut Procedure round just to be on the safe side.

My husband arrived at the hospital and, seeing me tapping, didn't interrupt. He stayed with me and I continued to tap, saying the Setups mentally. Occasionally, we talked and then I'd go back to tapping. After maybe another hour, I finally saw a doctor and I was still tapping. I told him I was doing EFT. He had never heard of it and I wasn't really up to explaining, so I made a mental note to send him some information about it later.

I still have some aches and pains from injured muscles and I've been tapping on them, individually and compositely. I have a thermopedic mattress topper so I was able to sleep comfortably even before I managed to remove all the pain aspects. I did take some Tylenol, but it was the tapping that made the difference. I wasn't able to breathe deeply due to a rib bruise, but I kept tapping and finally got some relief after thinking about the pain being like a strap around my chest. In fact, I pictured a thick brown belt with a silver buckle that I was opening so I could throw the belt away. Finally, when I was lying down, the tightness eased and I was able to breathe deeper. Of course, when I got up, many of the aches came back, but anyone could see that the healing was proceeding faster than usual.

All in all, I feel incredibly fortunate to have survived the accident—and even more fortunate to have a tool like EFT to work with anytime, anywhere, even under adverse conditions. Oh, and my husband has become a believer, too.

✿ ✿ ✿

Resources

Borrowing Benefits:
BorrowingBenefits.EFTUniverse.com

Choices Method by Patricia Carrington:
Choices.EFTUniverse.com

EFT for First Aid: TraumaTap.com

Movie Technique:
MovieTechnique.EFTUniverse.com

9 Gamut Procedure: 9Gamut.EFTUniverse.com

Practitioners: Practitioners.EFTUniverse.com

Tapping Circles: TappingCircles.EFTUniverse.com

Eliminating
Self-Sabotage

In any new project, there are several ways in which we can interfere with our own progress. By becoming familiar with these ways, you can recognize them when they appear and then use EFT tapping to remove them.

By far the easiest way to reach a goal is with the cooperation of your subconscious mind. If there's agreement or congruence between what your conscious mind wants and what your subconscious mind has been programmed to accept as possible, everything is likely to flow smoothly toward the goal. But if there's disagreement or incongruence, the conscious mind doesn't have a chance. In that situation, the subconscious mind always wins. Somehow circumstances will conspire to prevent you from reaching your goal, and the conscious mind will probably never understand what happened or why. It will simply forget about the project or attribute your failure to bad luck or circumstances. It won't realize that you, without being aware of it, prevented your own success.

If you have ever made a New Year's resolution regarding your health or physical fitness, you may understand this syndrome all too well. Your conscious mind really wants to get your body into shape and enjoy the benefits of physical fitness, and you may even start your new exercise program with enthusiasm. But a week later, you're back on the sofa watching television and eating potato chips.

If your back hurts, a vigorous exercise plan is probably the furthest thing from your mind, but it's a goal worth setting because the muscles that support your back, sides, and trunk work together to keep your back strong, flexible, and free from pain. As soon as you can, start walking, stretching, lifting weights, and doing exercises that build strength and stamina.

In addition, the combination of vigorous exercise and EFT is mutually reinforcing—exercise and the lymph circulation it stimulates make EFT more effective, and EFT enhances the positive effects of physical exercise.

Still, understanding this intellectually and embracing it emotionally are two different concepts. Do you resist exercising for reasons that have nothing to do with muscle spasms and pain? Sometimes the reasons for resisting are deeper than you think.

In the following article, certified EFT practitioner Carol Solomon, PhD, demonstrates how to get to these deeper issues of resistance and collapse them with EFT.

Using EFT to Overcome the
Resistance to Exercise

by Carol Solomon, PhD

My clients often develop resistance to exercise. They want to exercise, but either they don't feel motivated or don't enjoy it. They know they "should" exercise, but it can easily turn into an internal power struggle.

There can be other obstacles to overcome as well. Some women feel too embarrassed, ashamed, and/or self-conscious to go the gym at their current weight. So they avoid the activity that could actually help them lose weight. Others have perfectionist qualities; they think it won't make a difference, or it's not "worth it" unless they have time for a full 60-minute workout. So they don't go at all.

My client Susan wanted to talk about her resistance to going to the gym. She started out saying, "I love it… and I know I should do it, but it's not part of my routine… I need to make a plan." My intuition told me there was something deeper. I said, "Susan, it's not about planning." She said, "Why should I get excited or feel positive about anything? You know the other shoe is going to drop."

Two years ago, Susan's husband died while undergoing a routine sinus surgery. She pulled her life together and even began a new relationship. One week before this session, her new beau had been diagnosed with colon cancer. It was no wonder that Susan felt as she did.

Even though I don't want to get excited about anything because I know the other shoe is going to drop...

Even though nothing turns out right for me, I choose to move forward anyway.

Even though everything always gets messed up...

Eyebrow: *Why should I get excited?*

Side of Eye: *I know the other shoe is going to drop.*

Under the Eye: *Things never turn out right for me.*

Under the Nose: *Why bother?*

Chin: *I feel cursed.*

Collarbone: *It's not fair.*

Under the Arm: *I've tried so hard.*

Top of Head: *Everything always gets messed up.*

Susan was also worried that she wouldn't keep up her momentum. In the 2 years since her husband's death, she had had one crisis after another and couldn't follow through in her usual manner. Several attempts to make changes in her career got derailed when multiple crises occurred.

Even though I'm afraid I'll lose my momentum again... Even though I'm afraid I won't be able to maintain it...Even though I'm afraid something will happen, I choose to move forward anyway.

Eyebrow: *I've tried so hard.*

Side of Eye: *Everything's a crisis.*

Under the Eye: *I'm afraid something will happen.*

Under the Nose: *I'll just lose momentum again.*

Chin: *I won't be able to maintain it.*

Collarbone: *I'm not going to do it.*

Under the Arm: *You can't make me.*

Top of Head: *I don't want to be disappointed again.*

Eyebrow: *I choose to release these fears.*

Side of Eye: *I choose to move forward.*

Under the Eye: *I choose peace.*

Under the Nose: *I choose happiness.*

Chin: *I choose serenity.*

Collarbone: *I'm grateful for all the opportunities in my life.*

Under the Arm: *I choose to let it be fun and easy.*

Top of Head: *I can handle whatever comes.*

Since that session, which consisted of only two rounds of EFT, Susan began exercising with ease every day. She has also started a website and moved forward with significant changes in her career.

❀ ❀ ❀

Conditions That Interfere with Your Progress

Now let's consider some of the conditions that can interfere with your ability to reach the goals that you set. In addition to Psychological Reversal (see chapter 2), the following can also interfere: self-talk, tail-enders, and secondary gain (also discussed in Chapter 2). In the following sections, you will learn how to use EFT to resolve these interferences and move forward with your goals.

Self-Talk and the Writings on Your Walls

A potential stumbling block to reaching your goals with EFT is your subconscious mind and its programming, which is reflected in your self-talk: the thoughts and statements having anything to do with you that rattle around in your head at all hours of the day and night.

In EFT, the self-talk's programming is termed the "writings on your walls." This writing consists of all the "rules" you grew up with—statements you heard as a child, reflecting your family or cultural conditioning, and ideas or notions, especially about yourself, that you've absorbed throughout your life. Until you learn to tune in to your self-talk, you may be unaware of the "writings on your walls" that are governing you, your behavior, and who you're "allowed" to be in the world.

Here are some typical examples of these writings:

- It's hereditary. Back pain runs in my family.
- The doctor looked at my X-rays and said I'll never stop hurting. He's a doctor, he must be right.
- Everyone is used to me this way. This is how I'm supposed to be.
- I'll never get any better. I've been disappointed too many times. Nothing works for me.
- My job is here at home taking care of everyone. That's just how it is.
- My job is running a business to support my family. That's what I'm supposed to do.

Tail-Enders

Closely related to the writings on your walls are the tail-enders they inspire. Tail-enders are the "yes, but" statements that pop up when you try to set new goals or write new affirmations. The most obvious tail-enders are the words you hear in your mind when you try out a new idea. These words often have a sarcastic ring to them:

- Yeah, right.
- When pigs fly.
- I'll believe that when I see it.
- You must be kidding.
- Forget it.
- No way.
- Impossible.

Tail-enders are the nemeses of affirmations. A standard piece of advice in metaphysical circles is to turn negative self-talk around by stating the opposite. For example, if you hear yourself saying, "This is going to be a terrible day," try switching that to "This is going to be a wonderful day." If your conscious and subconscious minds accept the affirmation, it probably will be a wonderful day—but what if they don't? That's when tail-enders create mischief.

Tail-enders can show up at the end of a Choices statement, where you describe your goal, as in this example:

Even though this back pain is killing me, I choose to be completely free from pain and enjoy full range of motion...

…but I know that's never going to happen.

…but I really don't deserve to be well.

…but if I get well, I'm afraid my husband won't be as attentive and considerate as he is when I'm in pain.

…I'll have to go back to the job I hate.

…my daughter will be upset.

Secondary Gain

Many tail-enders reflect a problem called secondary gain. As discussed in chapter 2, secondary gain is a psychiatric term meaning that the person has a hidden or unconscious reason for holding onto an undesirable condition.

The term applies to chronic pain cases in which the patient will lose certain benefits if he or she gets well, such as attention from others, monetary compensation for disability, or the ability to keep denying the original cause of the pain. The subconscious mind feels more secure in the disadvantaged state than going for improvement.

So your conscious mind might be saying:

I sincerely want to get over this problem.

while your subconscious mind says:

I don't want to get over this problem because…

I can't ever get over this problem because…

It would be dangerous for me to get over this problem.

I can't afford to get over this problem.

What benefits do you receive from your back pain? Does keeping the pain feel safe? Does releasing it feel dangerous? Does keeping the pain generate sympathy from others that you won't receive if you're well? Does keeping the pain allow you to avoid unpleasant situations? Does keeping the pain give you financial rewards that you won't receive if you get well? Do you feel you don't deserve to be well? Do you fear that if you get well, something bad will happen?

I don't want to give up my back pain because...

...if I get completely well, I'll lose my disability payments and I'll have to get a job, and who knows how long that will take, and I've been unemployed for so long that I wouldn't know where to go or what to do, and the whole idea is just too stressful.

...if I get completely well, I'll have to move.

...my back pain is such an important part of my identity that I won't know who I'll be if it goes away.

...it's just too difficult.

Some short, effective Setup Statements that help neutralize the benefits of secondary gain include:

Even though I prefer to keep my back pain because _____, I deeply and completely accept myself anyway.

Even though part of me wants to stay sick, disabled, and incapacitated, I fully and completely accept myself.

Even though I like having this problem and intend to keep it and no one can make me give it up, so there, I nevertheless love and accept myself, I forgive and bless myself, I forgive my back, I forgive the part of me that keeps holding onto it, and I choose to facilitate the rapid healing of my back and all my emotions by releasing all my energy blocks beginning right now.

Using EFT to Overcome Self-Sabotage

A comprehensive Setup Statement can deal with all of these stumbling blocks—writings on your walls, tail-enders, and secondary gain issues, as well as Psychological Reversal—allowing you to reach your new goal with the full cooperation of your subconscious mind. Because it's important to release fears of not being able to cope or of being in danger if you let go of the pain, these Setup Statements can include safety nets, that is, reassurances that your brilliant subconscious mind can and will put you in the right place at the right time to bring benefits, not loss, into your life as you release the pain.

Here are some examples of Setup Statements to eliminate self-sabotage:

Even though I don't deserve to be completely well and free from pain, and I don't even want to get well, and I certainly don't deserve to get well, I choose to enthusiastically and creatively release all the guilt I used to feel about mistakes I made in the past.

Even though my back pain support group (or my friend Jane or my mom or my husband) will be upset if I get completely well and don't need their help anymore, I choose to enjoy my own excellent health and my own independent, happy life knowing that they will adjust and adapt just fine.

Even though if I get completely well, I won't be eligible for disability payments anymore, I welcome my perfect new job, which comes to me easily, comfortably, and with only good results.

Even though I have been receiving benefits from this back pain for a long time, I fully and completely accept myself. Even though I keep getting rewards for maintaining this back pain, I love and forgive myself. Even though this back pain prevents me from accomplishing my goals, and even though I may never let go of this back pain, I fully and completely accept myself, I love and forgive myself, I forgive my back, and I choose to be pleasantly surprised at how easy it is to instruct my subconscious mind to remove my attachment to any and all of the benefits and rewards that I receive or derive from maintaining this pain. I choose instead to receive rewards and benefits from releasing all of the pain in my back, opening myself to a new direction, and enjoying a new way of thinking and living. I choose to think and live in harmony with my goal of living a pain-free life beginning right now.

Of course, these statements are magnets for tailenders, writings on your walls, and other psychological interference. Your job is to continue treating them with EFT. Just notice what comes into your mind and keep tapping.

Saying Goodbye to the Past

Another way to release core issues that are related to past events and contribute to self-sabotage is to tap while saying:

Even though _____ happened, it doesn't have to cause pain in my back anymore. Even though _____ happened and I can't change the past, I can change my emotional connection to the past. Even though _____ happened, it doesn't affect me anymore, I can relax about it and let it go.

Using the tapping suggestions in this chapter, modifying the wording as needed to reflect the writings on your own walls and your particular circumstances, will help you put an end to the self-sabotage that is preventing your progress in eliminating your back pain with EFT.

Resources

Choices Method by Patricia Carrington:
Choices.EFTUniverse.com

Core Issues and How to Find Them:
CoreIssues.EFTUniverse.com

Tail-Enders: TailEnders.EFTUniverse.com

When Physical Symptoms Resist Healing:
SymptomsResistHealing.EFTUniverse.com

10

Improving Results

In some cases, EFT may be working very well without your realizing it. In others, success may follow a simple change of strategy. This chapter explores some common reactions in doing EFT and provides suggestions for dealing with them.

Chasing the Pain

One result that often confuses those new to EFT is that, with each round of tapping, their pain may find a new location, going from lower back to shoulder, from shoulder to neck, from neck to knee, and so on.

This moving pain may be evidence of changing emotional issues and a clue that at least one core issue is working its way toward the surface. As you relieve each pain with EFT tapping, you relieve the emotional issues behind it. Staying with the pain and tapping through all of its manifestations usually causes its gradual reduction and elimination, especially if you stop along the way to tap on any emotionally charged memories that come to mind.

An example of chasing the pain in EFT might go as follows:

> *Even though I have this sharp pointy arrow-like pain in my lower back...*
>
> *Even though the pain in my lower back has disappeared, I now have a throbbing hot orange ball of pain at the base of my neck...*
>
> *Even though I now have this small hard shiny black box of pain in my right hip...*
>
> *Even though I now have this dull aching pain in my right thigh...*
>
> *Even though I now have this sharp pointy red pain in my right knee...*

Approach each of these new locations as though it is a new pain, that is, with a new Setup Statement and tapping sequence.

In the next report, Marie LaForce, a registered nurse, describes how her client's pain moved from one location to another. This is a good example of how EFT's Basic Recipe did a thorough job of relieving pain. Because the pain eventually came back, exploring emotional issues that may be contributing to the pain and, for that matter, the overall condition (spinal stenosis) would be of further value.

Chasing Spinal Stenosis Pain

by Marie LaForce

I saw a woman who was in pain for the entire summer and wasn't sure why. This fall she was diagnosed with spinal stenosis, a narrowing of the spinal column that was putting pressure on her nerves. She had been seeing a physical therapist for about 3 weeks and was not getting much relief from her pain. I asked if she'd like to try EFT. She said, "Why not?"

We focused on the physical symptoms and began with her rubbing on the Sore Spot while saying:

> *Even though I have this pain in my left butt cheek, I deeply and completely accept myself.*

We followed the pain where it seemed most predominant (where she noticed it):

> *Even though I have this pain in my left hip...*
> *Even though I have this pain in my left knee...*
> *Even though I have this pain in my left thigh...*
> *Even though I have this pain in my left hip...*

We applied the entire Basic Recipe after each of the Setups, with no shortcuts. After tapping on "my hip" for the second time, she reported that the pain was gone. She got up and moved. The pain was still gone. As she sat on the couch, she told me that she generally wasn't able to sit for that length of time without feeling very uncomfortable. She had no pain at all when I left.

I called her a month later. She said the pain stayed away for about a week and gradually reappeared. When I talked to her, she was quite uncomfortable again. I believe that continued tapping on the pain or other issues such as support (problems with the spine) would have helped her to get at the additional aspects that were coming up.

❀ ❀ ❀

Mental Tapping

Instead of tapping with your fingers, try tapping with your imagination. This requires focus and concentration, but when you tune out everything else and really feel the connection, this method works very well.

Try a little mental tapping every day. Its obvious advantages are that it can be done anywhere at any time, it's totally discreet, it won't disrupt anything, and no one will realize you're doing anything unusual.

Some who try this method visualize themselves tapping as though they're watching themselves in a mirror.

Another way to tap mentally is to picture a laser light shining on the EFT point on which you are tapping in your mind. The laser light can be any color.

Still another approach is to imagine each EFT point pulsing or popping up on its own, like a button.

You can combine mental tapping with surrogate or proxy tapping (see the following section) to send balanced energy to others. As explained later in the chapter under "Borrowing Benefits," this technique will exert positive effects on your back pain, too.

When you try mental tapping for the first time, do it in a quiet location with no distractions. With practice, you'll be able to tap in your mind with good results even in noisy environments.

Surrogate or Proxy Tapping

In surrogate or proxy tapping, you tap on something else—usually yourself or a photo—in place of the person you hope to help.

EFT practitioners do proxy tapping all the time when they tap in person or by phone with clients for their clients' problems. Students attending EFT workshops do it whenever they tap along with someone whose problem is being treated onstage, the process called "Borrowing Benefits." Anyone who taps along with the videos on EFTUniverse.com does it, too. You will automatically do surrogate or proxy tapping whenever you work with a tapping buddy or with an EFT group.

Surrogate tapping can be used from any distance, from a few inches to thousands of miles. It can be done at any time, whenever you think of the person. However, a good ethical guideline to follow when surrogate or proxy tapping for someone is to get that person's permission before you tap. In the case of an infant, a mentally challenged individual, or anyone else who cannot understand and respond to the request, you would ask permission of the parent, guardian, or primary caretaker.

At the same time you are tapping for someone else, you can tap on yourself for your own emotional responses, especially for emotions like worry, frustration, impatience, guilt, anger, fear, grief, or depression.

You can also do surrogate tapping to help animals, including family pets, animals in zoos or on farms, and wild animals.

There are three basic ways to proceed in proxy or surrogate tapping. You can:

1. Tap as though you are the person or animal you want to help.

2. Tap as though you are talking to the person or animal you want to help.

3. Tap as though you are describing the person or animal you want to help.

For example, your friend Tom hurt his back playing baseball. If you're tapping with him in person, simply tap on yourself while saying his Setup Statements along with him as both of you tap together:

Even though I hurt my back sliding into second base, I fully and completely accept myself.

Even though I took a chance and it didn't pay off, I got tagged out and now my back is throbbing, I forgive and accept myself.

Even though it was dumb to try stealing bases at my age, I did what I did and now I choose to release all this pain in my back.

If you're by yourself and thinking about Tom, you can tap on yourself while using the same first-person Setup Statements, or you can use second-person Setups, as though you are talking to Tom:

Tom, even though you hurt your back sliding into second, I fully and completely accept you.

Even though you took a chance that didn't pay off, you got tagged out and now your back is throbbing, you can forgive and accept yourself.

Even though you're getting a little old to be stealing bases, the game is over, and now you can release all the pain in your back.

Or you can use third-person Setup Statements, as though you're talking about Tom:

Even though Tom hurt his back sliding into second, I fully and completely accept him.

Even though he took a chance that didn't pay off, he got tagged out and now his back is throbbing, he can forgive and accept himself.

Even though he's getting a little old to be stealing bases, the game is over, and now he can release all the pain in his back.

Borrowing Benefits

As noted in previous chapters, tapping on behalf of others can help clear your own back pain. This is one of the more unusual aspects of EFT. Every time you help someone else, you help yourself.

You can borrow benefits by tapping as you study this book, sending your energy to the people whose stories you're reading. You can borrow benefits by tapping as you watch EFT videos, or watch the news on television.

You can tap on behalf of people in magazines and online reports. You can tap on behalf of your boss, coworkers, customers, friends, neighbors, children, spouse, parents, other relatives, and people you've never met. Whenever you practice sending balanced energy their way, you'll feel better yourself. And if they're real people with real problems, your energy will make a difference in their lives as well.

You can do this tapping in person, such as while showing your brother-in-law how to relieve his sciatica, or from a distance (using surrogate or proxy tapping), or by phone.

Before you start tapping for others, select a problem of your own, focus on it for a moment, and then set it aside. While your conscious mind is busy tapping along for someone else, your subconscious mind will include your own situation in every tapping session.

The benefits you receive, or "borrow," don't have to relate in any way to the situations you tapped for. If your back is hurting, just focus for a moment on how it hurts, then give your undivided attention to the person you want to help. You can tap with a golfer to improve her swing, tap with a student to improve his grades, tap with a dieter about losing weight, or even tap for the family dog to help her indigestion—and all the while, your back will feel better.

In one EFT workshop, a man who owned a small business was stressed and distracted by a financial crisis that he didn't know how to resolve. He felt too over-whelmed to think straight. The instructor asked whether anyone in the group was in pain, and a woman asked for help with her menstrual cramps. Soon everyone in the room was tapping and saying, "Even though these cramps are killing me, I fully and completely accept myself." Two minutes later, the woman exclaimed that her cramps had completely disappeared—and the business-man excitedly announced, "While I was tapping about my menstrual cramps, I realized exactly how to fix my com-pany's problem."

Borrowing Benefits represents a big step in speed and efficiency in the delivery of EFT, producing, as it does, positive effects for a whole group of people tapping on only one person's problem.

The process also provides an additional measure of emotional safety. As you know, EFT is normally quite gentle, but a few people tune in to some intense emotional content and it can take awhile to lower their intensity ratings and remove the emotional charge. With the Borrowing Benefits feature, however, clients merely identify their issues and then tap along with someone else on an issue that is seemingly quite different. Thus a sort of detachment is injected into the process while the original issues are being addressed "in the background." In this way, it is like the Tearless Trauma Technique (see Chapter 5).

This way of defining and approaching problems helps to minimize any unwanted intensity while still getting the job done. The process may or may not give complete resolution to an issue but, properly done, it is likely to at least take the edge off, and probably much more. Very efficient, very useful, and very humane.

Borrowing Benefits is also a convenient way to get at core issues so that deep work can be done. An easy way to do this is to tap along with a video session of someone working on an issue that resembles your own. Here is an example of this from Melissa Derasmo.

Borrowing Benefits from DVD Session Eliminates Pain

by Melissa Derasmo

I had been struggling with severe neck and shoulder pain (always hovering around a level of intensity of 8 out of 10) for the last 6 months and had been tapping for it for the last 4 months with little to no improvement. I was quite convinced that this sharp pain fell into the impossible-to-fix category—until I watched a session with someone named Beth on an EFT training video.

As a habit, I tap along with every session on the DVDs, and this one was no exception. It appears that Beth's chronic pain was due in part to her issue of considering herself a savior—someone who needed to save everyone and fix the world. While this was not at all something I could identify with, I tapped along anyway. When the session was over, Beth's pain was gone—and so was mine!

This really shocked me. I had no idea that my wanting to fix everyone I met with EFT was, in fact, my way of playing the savior. I did quite a few rounds on every aspect I could come up with on this subject and the pain has yet to reappear—and I'm quite sure that it won't.

❈ ❈ ❈

Here is a suggestion from EFT Master Carol Look for Borrowing Benefits while watching television or movies: "I ask clients who watch a great deal of television or frequent movie theatres to tap for the characters' distress: 'Even though she feels insecure around that man...' 'Even though she won't admit the failure is her fault...' 'Even though he's afraid to confront the situation...' The clients do not have to identify their own issues first, just tap for the distress that their own system can't help but tune in to as a result of witnessing someone else's discomfort on the big screen."

You can even tap for the people in back pain commercials. This is a clever way of helping the subconscious mind neutralize some of the emotional charge connected to your own past events, making it easier to recognize, deal with, or simply release old problems. Tapping on behalf of fictional characters or real people you've never met brings you benefits, just as tapping on behalf of your best friend does.

Additional Tapping Procedures

You may not ever need the floor to ceiling eye roll, the Collarbone Breathing Exercise, or the 9 Gamut Procedure, but take a minute to become familiar with them so that you'll have them in your repertoire of EFT procedures. These techniques are both subtle and powerful, and they can trigger a breakthrough when progress seems to be stalled.

The Floor to Ceiling Eye Roll

This is a useful shortcut when you have brought the intensity of the problem down to a low level, such as to 1 or 2 on the 0-to-10 scale. It takes only 6 seconds to perform and, when successful, it will take you to 0 without you having to do another round of the Basic Recipe.

To perform it, simply repeat your Reminder Phrase while you tap the Gamut point continuously and, holding your head steady, take 6 seconds to move your eyes slowly from hard down to the floor to hard up to the ceiling. (For the location of the Gamut point, see chapter 3.)

Remember that this is an eye exercise, and your eyes are more likely to roll smoothly if they have something to follow. To provide this, hold both arms straight down in front of you. Keeping your head straight, lower your gaze to the floor. Begin tapping with one hand on the Gamut point of the other, and slowly raise both hands (keeping your elbows straight) until they are straight out in front of you, then continue moving them up until they are pointing straight at the ceiling. Follow your hand movement with your eyes throughout.

At the beginning of this eye exercise, while you face straight ahead, you won't be able to see either hand in their lowered position. As you slowly raise your hands, the fingertips of the tapped-on hand will move into view. Keep your eyes on the fingertips while your hand continues all the way up to the ceiling, at which point your fingertips will disappear from view again.

Reverse the direction and slowly bring your hands back down, following them with your eyes and tapping on the Gamut point all the while.

The Collarbone Breathing Exercise

In a few cases, a unique form of energy disorganization occurs within the body that impedes the progress of EFT. Its details are well beyond the scope of this book, but I *can* show you how to correct the problem. It is called the Collarbone Breathing Problem, not because there is something wrong with anyone's collarbone or breathing, but rather, it is named for its correction: the Collarbone Breathing Exercise. This correction was discovered by Dr. Roger Callahan, who developed Thought Field Therapy (TFT). The exercise need only be added when persistence with basic EFT is not showing results. It takes about 2 minutes to perform, and it may clear the way for the normal operation of otherwise impeded EFT procedures.

Here's how to do the Collarbone Breathing Exercise:

Although you can start with either hand, I'm going to assume you are starting with the right hand. Place two fingers of your right hand on your right collarbone point. You are going to be tapping on the Gamut point on that hand with the fingers of your left hand. Throughout the exercise, keep your elbows and arms away from your body so that the only things touching it are your fingertips and knuckles. Most people tend to drop their elbows, so remind yourself throughout to keep your elbows up, parallel to the floor, not touching your torso.

With two fingers of your left hand (keep your right elbow up), tap the right hand's Gamut point continuously while you perform the following five breathing exercises:

1. Breathe halfway in and hold it for seven taps.

2. Breathe all the way in and hold it for seven taps.

3. Breathe halfway out and hold it for seven taps.

4. Breathe all the way out and hold it for seven taps.

5. Breathe normally for seven taps.

Place the two fingers of your right hand on your *left* collarbone point and, while continuously tapping the right hand's Gamut point, do the five breathing exercises.

Next, bend the fingers of your right hand so that the second joint or "knuckles" are prominent. Place these knuckles on your right collarbone point and tap the right hand's Gamut point continuously while doing the five breathing exercises.

Repeat this with the right knuckles placed on the left collarbone point.

You are now halfway through the collarbone breathing exercise. You complete it by repeating the entire procedure using the fingertips and knuckles of the *left* hand. You will be tapping the left hand's Gamut point with the fingertips of the right hand.

If you have used EFT persistently and your results are either slow or nonexistent, start each round of basic EFT with the Collarbone Breathing Exercise. You may find that it "clears the way" and allows dramatic relief.

Resources

Borrowing Benefits:
    BorrowingBenefits.EFTUniverse.com

Choices Method by Patricia Carrington:
    Choices.EFTUniverse.com

Collarbone Breathing:
    CollarboneBreathing.EFTUniverse.com

Core Issues and How to Find Them:
    CoreIssues.EFTUniverse.com

Floor to Ceiling Eye Roll: FTC.EFTUniverse.com

Tail-Enders: TailEnders.EFTUniverse.com

When Physical Symptoms Resist Healing:
    SymptomsResistHealing.EFTUniverse.com

11

Pain, Anger, and Metaphors

By now you understand how EFT can be used to relieve back pain and every other kind of pain. You have progressed beyond the basic protocol and are well on your way to EFT artistry.

At this point, I'd like to return to Dr. Sarno's theory of back pain—that your back hurts because you're angry—and focus on using EFT as a tool for forgiving, forgetting, and letting go of anger. Given that anger is a factor in so many people's back pain, this is an important area for you to explore on your healing journey.

The first step is to consider the words and phrases you use unconsciously and habitually that may be setting you up for and entrenching back pain.

Metaphors and Back Pain

Metaphors are colorful words or phrases that we use as analogies to describe things, people, and situations. They can be entertaining and expressive, but psychologists warn that our bodies take all of the words we use seriously. Consider this common statement:

She's such a pain in the neck.

If you refer to someone in your life as a "pain in the neck" long enough or often enough, guess what? You can wind up with an actual pain in your neck.

That is why skilled EFT practitioners ask their pain clients questions like:

Who's stuck in your spine?

Who is the pain in your neck?

What's the heavy weight that you're carrying?

Who stabbed you in the back?

Think of what your body might do with some common expressions such as:

My back is killing me.

This pain is driving me crazy.

By paying attention to the images contained in our language and eliminating ones with detrimental associations, such as the previous, we can prevent our bodies from interpreting images as instructions that end up being damaging to our health and well-being. The following report by Gary Clark demonstrates this principle.

Clearing a Back Pain Metaphor

by Gary Clark

After watching EFT on video extensively, I decided to start using EFT in my practice. I am a myotherapist so I deal mainly with people's muscle pain.

When a new patient arrived to have her back pain treated, I was surprised to find that she didn't have much in the way of the trigger points that usually cause this type of pain.

After I dealt with the few soft-tissue problems I could find, her pain level fell from a 10 to an 8.

"Okay," I said, "can you point to the exact place where it hurts?"

She indicated the top of the sacrum. I placed my hand there and said, "If this part of your back could talk to you, what would it say?"

Quick as a flash she said, "Escape."

"And what do you want to escape from?"

"Work," she replied.

"And what is it about work that you want to escape from?"

"Oh," she said, "I run my own business, and work has been terribly slow lately. It's a real pain in the butt."

"Did you hear what you just said?" I asked.

"Oh, my God," she exclaimed, "I've been telling everyone for the last 3 weeks that work is a pain in the butt."

I grinned and said, "Be careful what you wish for. You just might get it."

I quickly taught her EFT and we did two rounds of tapping on:

> *Even though I have been saying that work is a pain in the butt, I truly and deeply accept myself.*

Those two rounds completely cleared the pain. Later, I couldn't help thinking that I could have saved us both a lot of time if I had used EFT right away.

❖ ❖ ❖

Here's a fascinating report from EFT Universe Trainer Dale Teplitz about how literal the mind can be when it generates pain.

Shooting Back Pain—an Amazing Metaphor
by Dale Teplitz

Metaphors often crop up while doing EFT. I find them of great value in providing clues to the cause of physical and emotional pain. Sorting through the metaphors and all their possible meanings is often well worth the effort. Metaphors can provide examples of how we literally store trauma and experiences in our body's energy system. The EFT practitioner can be of value by noticing the metaphor and taking the client in that direction. Here is a stunning example in which the client identified her own metaphor.

Betty attended a Level 2 EFT workshop that I taught in Los Angeles in March 2006. When I asked whether anyone had a difficult physical symptom they would like to work on in front of the group, Betty volunteered. She had been trying to rid herself of low back pain for years. She suggested that it was a really tough one! Nothing she tried had worked. She was stumped about the relationship between this pain and any particular emotions.

As she bravely ascended the podium to work with me, Betty reported having a sharp pain that ran from her lower back to her right foot. Her doctor called it sciatica.

Betty is a very bright, articulate, and introspective woman in her 60s who has been a marriage and family therapist for over 20 years. She spent much of her adult life as a tireless seeker of healing for her own childhood wounds as well as those of her clients.

Her life was filled with struggles, which began at the moment of her own birth, a traumatic C-section. Many serious challenges involving family relationship issues followed.

When Betty was a vulnerable 14 years old, her father took his own life. At that moment, her childhood ended. She was forced to become the "parent" to her mother. Her young life was filled with burden.

In the workshop, we began tapping about her back pain with the basic EFT recipe. While tapping, I encouraged her to describe the pain in increasingly specific ways. When I asked how the pain moved, she reported that it "shot" from her lower back to the large toe of her right foot.

As she traced the pain with her hand to demonstrate to us where it was, her jaw dropped. In this "light bulb" moment, Betty remembered that when her father ended his life, he tied a shoelace from the big toe of his right foot to the trigger of the shotgun he used to shoot himself in the head. He was literally "shooting from the toe!"

All of us, including Betty, were astonished at the unfolding metaphor. By the look on her face, she had no doubt about the connection between the shooting pain to her toe and her father's death. Betty and I began to unravel the metaphor as we tapped each point.

This shooting pain. This shooting toe pain. Dad shooting himself in the head pain...

For every thought and memory she expressed, we tapped. Layers of deep trauma, shame, and grief welled up and were collapsed with EFT within minutes. They were gradually replaced with compassion for what she and her father had been through. The shooting pain disappeared. Betty looked lighter!

Eighteen months later, Betty reports that the shooting pain has not returned. Although now retired from counseling, Betty continues to use EFT as an important piece to the healing puzzle for herself, her family, and her friends.

❊ ❊ ❊

The next report illustrates how quickly a well-timed question can stop pain. When Gillian Wightman's son complained of a stabbing pain between his shoulder blades, one question got to the heart of the matter.

She Stabbed Him in the Back

by Gillian Wightman

Two years ago, my son, who was then 16, had an acute stabbing pain in his back. He resisted the idea of using EFT for the pain, arguing that it was a physical problem that needed manipulation. My husband and I are trained in craniosacral therapy, so I knew I had the skills to treat him if this was the case.

However, I also knew that this pain had started when it became clear things had changed between him and a girl he had had a crush on for years. They had not embarked on a relationship but had an understanding, and one night at a group event she treated him very badly. I think it was her clumsy way of letting him know her feelings had changed that hurt him so much. The pain appeared the next day.

When he came begging for help with his back, I got him to lie on the couch and I put my hands under his back, where the pain was, right between the shoulder blades. I asked him how the pain felt and he described it as if a knife was stabbing into his back. I waited a little and then asked, "So who stabbed you in the back?"

He shouted out, "Becky!" Then he said, "Oh, you got me, didn't you? How do you do that?" He was laughing and he agreed to try EFT. We worked through all his feelings of frustration and confusion. She wouldn't talk to him and he had no idea what had happened or what he had done wrong. There were a lot of very painful emotions in his back. We started with:

Even though Becky stabbed me in the back…

and that immediately brought his pain from a 10 down to a 2 or 3. We then fine-tuned it by tapping for different aspects of his anger, hurt, and confusion. Tapping through all of his heartbreak totally relieved this acute pain and I am happy to say he now enjoys a good platonic relationship with this girl.

❁ ❁ ❁

Letting Go of Anger

If the healing process has a main theme, it could be forgiveness. EFT will work even if you hold onto grudges, but it works better if you let them go. After all, grudges and anger are disturbing emotions, and disturbing emotions are a contributing factor in physical pain.

Occasionally, someone demonstrates just how powerful the connection between these held emotions and physical pain is. Consider what happened to Caroline, who worked for many years as a school bus driver. Two years ago, her school van was rear-ended by a truck in an accident that left her with painful injuries.

Caroline attended an EFT training class 7 months after the accident, not because she was interested in the subject but because she was delivering something for the instructor. As long as she was there, she decided to tap along with the group and she was soon startled to realize that over 70% of her chronic pain from the accident had spontaneously disappeared. "I can't believe it," she exclaimed. "This stuff works better than 7 months of physical therapy!"

Soon the whole class was tapping with her, focusing on the accident, the school van, the pain, the 7 months of physical therapy, and the frustration of being injured. Caroline kept feeling better and better. In fact, her pain completely disappeared—until the instructor had everyone say, "I completely forgive the man who rear-ended my van."

While the rest of the class continued tapping, Caroline froze. Her eyes grew wide with that deer-in-the-headlights look, she couldn't move and, as soon as the round was over, she complained, "Now the pain is worse than it was before."

Despite understanding that there was a clear connection between her unforgiveness and her pain, Caroline found it impossible to let go of her anger toward the other driver. As she told the class, "I can't forgive him. That's God's job. If God wants to forgive him, that's fine, but it's not my job."

With a great deal of coaxing, she was eventually able to say something far less threatening. She tapped and said:

Even though I can't forgive the guy who crashed into me, I would like to consider the possibility of perhaps one day, some day, maybe forgiving him just a little.

That was at least a tiny step in the right direction, but more than that she refused to consider.

Still, the message got through, and every day Caroline's body reminded her of the pain that unforgiveness can cause. A large black sun just to the right of her shoulder blade shot painful black rays into her back and shoulder, interfering with her sleep, exercise, and every other aspect of her life. Caroline understood intellectually that the pain was linked to her anger, and she tried through prayer and meditation to release it, but without success. When she became sufficiently desperate, she asked the EFT instructor for help.

Caroline was soon combining EFT with Dr. Carrington's 1% solution (see Chapter 12). She focused on her anger and frustration toward the man who was her boss at the time of the accident because he refused to call an ambulance, insisting that she didn't need medical attention. She drove herself to her own doctor, who believed her brain was bleeding and sent her to an emergency room where she was treated for multiple injuries.

At the time of the accident, while she waited at a red light behind other vehicles, Caroline had a split second before impact in which to turn the wheel so that her van didn't crash into the car in front of her. Instead of being applauded for preventing death or injury to others, she was blamed for causing the accident. Workers' compensation bureaucrats denied her claim while making false accusations and repeatedly misplacing her proof of injury.

Caroline had many legitimate grievances, but as she tapped, vented, and occasionally cried, her dark cloud of anger, frustration, and unforgiveness lifted, and she was soon saying, "It was just an accident. It's over. And thanks to being laid off, I went back to school, took classes that I would never have been able to take, completed my training as an emergency medical technician, and am enrolled in a PhD program. If it weren't for the accident, I would never have been able to do these things." Note the cognitive shift here. For almost 2 years, Caroline had repeated her story to anyone who would listen with the same words and the same story line. Suddenly her perspective shifted and she looked at it entirely differently.

By the end of her 20-minute session, Caroline was enthusiastically tapping to release not just 1% of her anger and unforgiveness, but rather all of it, and she was laughing, rejoicing, sighing, stretching, and thoroughly enjoying her new pain-free life. In the 2 months that followed, she reported ever-increasing freedom from pain, improved range of motion, and growing happiness and optimism.

At an EFT workshop for therapists, some of the attending therapists brought their "tough clients" for the instructors to work with. One was a middle-aged woman who had been in several automobile accidents 2 years prior. She reported that she had a metal plate in her neck and that her right arm was beset with pain that was always at a 9 or 10. And she meant *always*. It never let up.

Two rounds of basic EFT on her arm pain produced no result. Then the instructor asked her: "If there was an emotional contributor to this pain, what would it be?"

The woman didn't hesitate, letting loose in an angry tirade about the driver of the car that hit her, the incompetence of her physicians, and on and on. There was nothing subtle about her anger. Her face turned red and the veins stood out in her neck.

Two or three rounds—about two minutes total—of tapping on the anger dissipated the anger. She then spoke of the incident in much calmer terms, and the pain in her arm had dropped to 0. Two months later, her therapist reported that the woman's arm pain had remained at a 0.

Anger is one of those emotions that can help us or harm us. In fairness to anger, it can motivate us to act in order to change harmful situations, but most of the time it just festers or causes new problems. Fortunately, once we uncover anger, it's easy to treat and transform with EFT.

Dr. El March provides another example of using EFT to identify and release anger issues involved in back pain.

Severe Back Pain Subsides
After Anger Issue Uncovered

by Dr. El March

I've been in the field of orthomolecular medicine for many years, so when Ed came to me for lower back pain after 3 months of not being able to go to work or move in any direction, we tried a number of things in an effort to get him up and running.

I sent him to chiropractors, had him do exercises, and put him on megavitamin therapy, only to have him return with severe pain every few months and later every few years. This year Ed came to my office completely stiff and in great pain, looking for more exercises and advice to ease the situation. This time I decided to try the EFT method on him and with his permission we started.

I knew that he had been suffering from this problem for more than 10 years. I first did three rounds of basic EFT and tapped with him for the pain, which went from a 10 to 5 and back up to 10 again.

We started talking and I learned he had been laid off from his job a couple of years back and is now in business for himself. His business is stressful and he cannot afford to take the time off.

So we tapped for:

> *Even though this pain is the only way that I can rest and spend some time at home without feeling guilty that I'm not making any income…*

We also tapped on:

> *Even though I don't believe this method is going to do anything for me…*

During these rounds of tapping, the pain dropped to an 8 and then to a 5, but no matter how many more rounds we did, it stayed stuck, going back and forth between 5 and 8.

Then I asked Ed to explain his emotions toward the pain and he said, "Anger." He went on to tell me the story of how his back pain had come about:

"I was employed at a financial institution as a senior computer center analyst. On the day this happened, I was monitoring the progress on a job I had given one of my staff to do when some computers were delivered to our laboratory. As I was looking for someone to set the computers up, my manager, Dan, walked in and asked me to haul the computers to a different location in the lab where they were waiting for installation.

"I felt his action was uncalled for and disrespectful to my seniority and grade level. This was completely out of line and not part of my functions, and I felt belittled in front of the employees who reported directly to me. As I was lifting one of the boxes, the muscle in my back made a noise and I felt heat rushing through my lower back. I couldn't move after that. I was sent home and stayed on short-term disability for about 3 months. I first came to see you 1 month before I went back to work."

After hearing this explanation, I decided to tap with Ed on the feelings he had going back to 1994 and his manager's actions:

Even though my manager was disrespectful to me and belittled me in front of my staff and I don't believe he had the right to ask me to do what he did, I completely and lovingly accept myself, I love and respect myself, I forgive myself and I forgive Dan.

Once we finished tapping on this, the pain dropped from 8 to 3. Ed kept calling Dan an ass, so I did another round of tapping on:

> *Even though Dan behaved like a complete ass and was completely out of line for asking me to move the computers, I completely and lovingly accept myself. I love and forgive myself and I forgive Dan.*

Two rounds of EFT and Ed's pain was completely gone. He was amazed and did not believe it would last. I checked with him the next day, the next week, and again a few months later. The pain had still not returned.

I think EFT has added quite an edge to my regular practices. I have used it on myself and family members to quickly treat shoulder pain, headaches, nausea, and so on. This method is absolutely invaluable.

❈ ❈ ❈

In the next article, Kaye Bewley describes how a client who had suffered from lower back pain for 25 years and upper back pain for 4 years finally found relief—from an hour-long session of EFT. Key to the resolution of the pain was release of long-held anger. Notice how Kaye handled the core issue, which her client did not want to express.

Anger and Rage Are at the Root of This Back Pain

by Kaye Bewley

When Alison arrived on my doorstep, her face was creased with a deep, furrowed frown. She had the look of someone who had been in pain for a long time and had come to accept it as a burden. Alison said she had been plagued with a pain in her upper back for about 4 years and pain in her lower back for the past 25 years.

Recently, she had taken drugs for the pain and, unfortunately, reacted very badly to them. She had even had to be admitted to the hospital's coronary ward because they thought she was having a heart attack. She said it felt as though a tight band had been drawn across her chest. Also, the weekend prior to seeing me, she had been doing some exercises and strained her shoulder so badly that she couldn't raise her arm.

She wondered whether EFT would be able to do something for her as she had already spent over £2,000 on alternative therapies that hadn't worked.

We sat down and concentrated on the pain in her back, which she rated at an 8. After one round, it went down slightly to 7, so we completed another couple of rounds, one with negative statements such as:

I don't want to release this pain in my back.

and the next with positive statements such as:

I may consider releasing this pain in my back.
I can choose to be without this pain in my back.

After completing these rounds, she rated the pain as going down to a 5, and for the first time in a long time, she smiled.

Another few rounds concentrated on the pain in her back, after which we tentatively began to explore the emotional issues that might be behind it.

Alison mentioned that her social life was okay, but she admitted to having some problems at work, such as having to cover for everyone who had been off sick and feeling as though she couldn't let the company down. She had recently been verbally abused by a customer without any support from her boss, who witnessed the situation. She had also been given extra tasks which were beyond her physical capabilities. We went through another round of tapping on specific issues related to these instances, and finally came to the crux of her pain—anger.

She began to explore some problems she had been experiencing with a manipulative, inconsiderate step-brother. He had upset one of her friends with his cheating and lies, and she felt very hurt by that.

She said there were many scenes that gave rise to the angry feelings inside, but when I asked her to describe one, she said she didn't want to express it. This was okay, as in EFT, the therapist doesn't need to know all the details of your emotional experiences. We simply picked a word that related to the scene and concentrated on that.

Thus a "rage" rating of 8 was decided upon and we tapped on the EFT points. Three rounds of tapping brought her anger levels down from 8 to 7½, then to 5, then to 2.

Alison then mentioned a couple of long-standing issues that were coming into focus about her stepbrother. She felt angry because he wasn't supportive of her parents when they became ill. Her rage at him in that particular situation was higher than a 10, but after tapping for several rounds, we managed to bring it down to a 3, which was wonderful.

At this point, we took a well-earned breather and I explained how the words of others condition our thoughts. I gave a few examples, but none of them fit with her until I asked her if she had ever been told by her parents not to leave the table until she had finished her meal.

Aha! She said her mum always made her sit at the table and finish her vegetables and threatened her with not being able to have her pudding if she didn't eat all of her main meal.

She found the funny side of this as we tapped on it, using it as a metaphor for the way things kept happening in her life now. We found a pattern in that she always had to work hard before she was able to get any pleasure in life, but she ended up not getting any pleasure after all because she there was always something she had to do before she was able to relax.

Now she found herself working hard under the management of a boss who didn't stand up for her and under the direction of supervisor who made her do work she wasn't able to keep up with physically, on top of which she had to take care of her parents and deal with her stepbrother.

She tapped while saying:

Even though I care for people and am able to help them through difficulties, I may consider having a little bit of fun for myself as well.

Even though I don't feel supported by anyone, and this is showing up as a pain in my back, I can accept and love all of me and deserve some pleasure in life.

Even though I feel as though I have to work all the time without enjoying any pleasures, I know it doesn't have to be like this, I can have my cake and eat it, too.

We decided to wind the session down at that point. After 60 minutes of tapping, Alison said that her feelings of rage had lessened a lot and that the pain in her back and shoulder had reduced. She also said that after all the money she had spent on alternative therapies over the past few years, she had never experienced as much relief as she had with EFT. Best of all, the EFT worked in a remarkably short space of time!

A few weeks later, Alison reported that she was quite happy with the way the session had gone and that her back was much more comfortable. She added that she received a pleasant side effect of feeling calmer than she had ever felt in her life.

✿ ✿ ✿

As long as your subconscious mind has a reason for holding onto anger, it can be difficult if not impossible to dissolve. A leading reason for retaining anger and unforgiveness is the notion that if we forgive someone for something unforgivable, we're condoning what he or she did. Worse, we're encouraging that person to repeat the action or do something worse.

When It's Impossible to Forgive

by Cathleen Campbell

Often the concept of forgiveness is distasteful or seemingly impossible because it conveys a sense that what the offender did would be accepted or allowed without an apology, or that forgiveness would somehow signal to the offender that he or she could repeat the offense. We want the people who hurt us to acknowledge that pain, to convey their deep sorrow, and finally convince us that they will never again put us in such misery.

Because our feelings are so strong, we believe we must be right and, if we can't be right, then not only must we be wrong, but our pain would then be wrong, too. In such a state, it's impossible to see that both parties could actually be right, or that perhaps there's some gray area in which no one is fully wrong. To comprehend and acknowledge all of this while in an acute state of pain is simply too much to bear.

When we suspend judgment and simply tap for release, however, all sorts of new and interesting ideas begin to come to the surface. Since we are not asking ourselves to agree that something horribly wrong is now miraculously okay, our guard doesn't go up as firm and fast.

Shifting from the unproductive cycle of "they're wrong and I'm right" allows us to release our feelings of injustice. Sometimes the shifts can be so quick and dramatic that instead of maintaining the pain or grudge, a sense of understanding redefines the entire problem and we end up seeing the offender as the real victim!

Most often, though, asking our subconscious to help our conscious mind with understanding gives us new insights that allow us to dissolve the pain slowly. Even better, it helps us create new tactics with which to handle the situation. In situations that are ongoing, such as having to be around an offensive coworker or a family member, bringing new understanding into the equation gives us a new perspective from which to create the new reality we so dearly wish to live.

❊ ❊ ❊

The following report from EFT practitioner Stefan Gonick expands on the issue of subconsciously not wanting to let go of anger because that would mean the offender got away with the offense. He illustrates how he cleared these hidden beliefs with a client. You may find the tapping language he uses helpful for your own work on anger.

Letting Go of Anger That Feels Necessary

by Stefan Gonick

I worked with three clients recently who had anger issues for which EFT tapping didn't initially help much at all. In each case, the person was angry about a serious offense that happened a very long time ago. There was nothing to be done or even said to the offending person, and in one case the offender had died. These clients were aware that the offenders from long ago were not being affected at all by their anger and that they were the only ones suffering. However, neither these realizations nor EFT relieved their anger.

When this happened with the first client, we were stuck for a while, but then I had a flash of intuition. I asked my client whether she felt that letting go of her anger would mean that the other person would somehow "get away with" what he did. A light bulb went on in her mind and she agreed.

She subconsciously felt that her anger was, in a cosmic justice sort of way, keeping the other person "accountable" for what he did. She was afraid that if she let go of her anger, it would mean that what he did to her "didn't matter" and he would "get away with it" without any consequences. The dilemma was that she herself was the only person actually being affected by her anger, but it felt as though letting go of it would be to his benefit. So we tapped on:

Even though he'll get away with what he did if I don't stay angry...

Even though he won't be accountable without my anger...

Even though my anger matters regarding what he did to me...

Later in the tapping we included affirming phrases like:

> *I release him to the Universe.*
>
> *He is subject to his own karma.*
>
> *I choose peace for myself.*

After several rounds of this nature, my client's anger disappeared and she felt great relief and peace around the issue.

After encountering this same situation with the next two clients in a row, I felt that this insight might be helpful to others, and it was. So, if you find yourself having a hard time relieving your anger through tapping, look deeper within to see if issues of "cosmic justice" are getting in your way.

✦ ✦ ✦

Australian EFT practitioner Angie Muccillo describes an EFT exercise that has widespread uses. The basic idea is to tap while you listen to your body in a unique way and let it tell you about the real issues underlying your back pain. Along the way, you may discover metaphors that make core issues obvious or that help you understand just where your anger, discomfort, dissatisfaction, frustration, and pain are really coming from. If you haven't ever had a meaningful two-way conversation with your body, now's the time to begin.

What Your Aching Body Has to Say

by Angie Muccillo

You complain about your body—that damn shoulder, those bung knees, your sore back, that creaky neck—but how about giving your body a chance to complain about you? I wonder what it would have to say.

The purpose of this exercise is to give your painful body parts a chance to voice their point of view and express their pain and hurt while giving you a chance to really listen and take note. In this exercise, you will be paying attention to your aching, screaming body parts. This is an exercise in "in-tuition" or learning from within. It involves tuning in to your body and learning what it needs by listening to how it feels.

Communicating with your body in this way can reestablish or strengthen your connection to it. Sometimes we spend so much time complaining about our pain (either silently or aloud) that we forget to stop and listen for the message in the pain. Once we understand what our shoulder is angry about, for example, we can release it with EFT.

Let's see what a typical shoulder has to say. If you have a shoulder complaint of any sort, do your shoulder a favor and tap along. Simply tap the EFT points continuously as you read this script and borrow the benefits from this shoulder complaint. This is one uptight shoulder!

A Word from Your Shoulder Complaint

Hi, it's me, your shoulder. Yes, that's right. Remember me? It's nice to be heard, *finally!* Where do I begin? I've tried and tried to get your attention over and over again, but you just won't listen to me. I have sent you repeated pain signals and messages, but you ignore all my warnings and push on despite them. What's that all about? I don't understand why I have to get so red and angry to be heard. It's the only time you acknowledge me — and when you do, all I get is condemned. "That damn shoulder!" you cry. I feel like hunching over every time you hurl abuse at me. How do you think that makes me feel?

You complain about me. Well, you know what? I've got a few complaints of my own. I've been carrying your load and burdens all these years, and what sort of appreciation do I get? *None!* To be honest, I am fed up and angry with you for treating me so badly. I've been supporting you all these years but I'm cracking and crumbling under the pressure. All I want is to know that I am doing a good job. Just the slightest acknowledgment would do. Some positive attention for a change would be greatly appreciated.

Butyou keep saying yes when you mean no. I'm sick and tired of it. I wish you would follow your nos for a change. But because you don't follow your nos, you always end up overcommitting yourself and working too long and too hard and you don't even enjoy it most of the time. Then you take it all out on me and complain incessantly about how I bother you and what a pain I am and how I stop you from doing what you need to do. I just tighten up more and more every time I hear you say yes to something you don't want to do or be or have. I'm sick and tired of being tied up in knots all the time!

If you insist on carrying all those burdens and don't learn to say no when you mean no, then I'm going to have to say it for you by flaring up and firing a few more pain signals your way. I might even freeze right up so you can't move and then you'll be forced to stop what you are doing right there and then. I know that may seem a little harsh, but that way you might get the message that I'm overworked and overtired and deserve a holiday! Here's the deal. I'll rush you a load of those feel-good chemicals you like so much, just as soon as you relax and give me a break! Deal?

How to Take Note of Your Complaints

Here are step-by-step guidelines for writing your own script for listening to your body:

Step 1. Choose a physical complaint, and ask your complaint to state its own complaints.

Step 2. Invite your aching body part to speak up. Ask for the loudest complaint to come forward and deal with this one first.

Step 3. Focus on the area of your body you would like to heal—shoulder, neck, back, stomach—and ask it to tell you how it feels. Encourage your chosen body part to express any complaints and upsets openly and honestly and without holding back. Listen carefully and write down everything you are being told, take note of every complaint, every unheard request and every upset. You are at the service of your body here. Your job is simply to take note. Allow yourself to be creative in the process.

Step 4. Once you have finished your script, read it aloud and either tap continuously on the EFT points or rub the Sore Spot until you get to the end of the script. Then use a Reminder Phrase at each point, such as *"this (name of body part) complaint."*

Step 5. Write a reply to your complaint in the form of a Self-Care Plan. This is your chance to address your body's complaints. Write to your complaint or simply talk to it about your intentions to address its concerns. You may want to start by acknowledging its complaints and showing empathy for what it is experiencing. You can then explain what you plan to do (what action you will take) to address these complaints. For example, a Self-Care Plan for the previous shoulder complaint might sound something like the letter that follows. Again, tap along to borrow the benefits as you read.

Dear Shoulder — Yes, I hear you loud and clear now that I've stopped and taken time out of my busy schedule to take note of how you feel about all this. I know I've been a pain to live with lately, but things are going to change now. Even though in the past I was guilty of not listening to you, from now on I vow to tune in to how you are feeling and do what is necessary to take care of it. As soon as I start to receive a pain signal from you, I will promise to stop and look at what I'm doing that is overloading you. I vow to take care, respect, praise, and appreciate you for your hard work.

Yes, you have carried me all this time and now I take the time to show my appreciation. How's this—I will ensure that you get a massage at least once a fortnight, or weekly if your complaining gets too loud. I will take your advice and start saying no when I mean no. *Even though I've been guilty of saying yes when I mean no, I choose to follow my nos from now on.* I will take a long hard look at what I take on and whether it is in my best interests. I put you first and focus on getting balance back into my life, so you don't have to work so hard. Hey, and guess what! I just went to see the boss and I've put in for 6 weeks off. Now does that sound like a Self-Care Plan or what?

If you have difficulty tuning in to your body and you can't "hear" the messages, try these little EFT tune-ups:

Even though I can't tune in to what my body is trying to tell me, I choose to listen for the message in the pain.

Even though I'm so out of touch with my body's needs, I choose to practice listening and taking note of what my body is trying to tell me.

Even though until now I have neglected and ignored the messages from my body, I choose to pay more attention from now on.

The more you take note of your body's complaints and tap on these complaints, the less likely it is that your body will complain at all. You can apply this process to all your physical complaints, starting with the loudest ones first.

Using this technique regularly may lead to pain reduction. It can also be used in a preventative manner by helping you stay in tune with your body and giving it what it needs for optimum health, whether it is better nutrition, more rest, more exercise, recovery time, letting go of certain obligations, cutting back work hours, increasing recreation time, increasing creative pursuits, or other factors that are there, in your body, waiting to be discovered.

❊ ❊ ❊

Here are some innovative approaches to chronic pain by Sangeeta Bhagwat from India. These same ideas can be useful for a wide variety of ailments.

EFT and Skillful Metaphors for Rheumatoid Arthritis Pain

by Sangeeta Bhagwat

I have been working with Mrs. J for her rheumatoid arthritis (RA) symptoms. RA pain is constant and terrible. As she had tried several allopathic (conventional) and Ayervedic (traditional Indian) medicines over the years, her homeopath asked her to avoid taking any medicines for about 15 to 20 days, to allow her body to detoxify. She continued her painkillers and a sleeping pill.

One day, her pain was highly unbearable, so she asked me to try EFT. She was complaining of severe pain in her shoulders. I first did one round, using:

> *Even though I have this unbearable pain in my shoulders, I deeply and completely love, forgive, and accept myself.*

She reported a reduction in her level of intensity from 8 to 7½ out of 10. I then asked her to describe the pain, asking her whether it had a color or texture. She replied that it was dark gray and like a sticky liquid.

So I started tapping on her with the following Setup:

> *Even though I have this dark grey, sticky pain weighing down my shoulders, I choose to drain it away.*

While I was tapping, I told her to imagine a tube draining away this pain, while she repeated *"Drain away"* at each point. Two rounds reduced her level of intensity to 2 out of 10.

I asked her to describe the pain again. She said it was now dark and thick. So while tapping at the Karate Chop point, we used:

> *Even though I have this stubborn, dark, and sticky pain in my shoulders, I apply heat to it so that it becomes thinner and can drain away easily. I drain away this remaining pain.*

The pain subsided. I worked on some more underlying emotional issues and gave her homework rounds to do.

After a few days, she again called with severe shoulder pain. When asked to describe it, she called the pain "four huge boulders." So I used:

>*Even though these four heavy boulders are weighing me down, I choose to break them with a laser gun.*

That did not work, so I changed it to:

>*Even though these four boulders are weighing me down, I choose to hammer them to pieces,*

with "hammer" as the Reminder Phrase. Immediately, she felt that the boulders had shattered to pieces and the pain had "rolled away."

She then stood up with some difficulty and said that the pain had dropped to around her hips. When asked to describe it, she said it was like a string of heavy rocks around her hip. So I used:

>*Even though I have this money belt of painful rocks around my hips, I deeply and completely love, forgive, and accept myself.*

There was only a marginal movement in her level of intensity. I felt that she was reluctant to let go of the pain, so I changed the Setup to:

>*Even though this pain is terrible, I don't want to change. I am used to it and don't want to let go.*

After tapping one shortcut round of this, I changed the Setup to:

>*Even though I don't want to let go of these 10 rocks I have around my hips, perhaps I could let go of just one.*

After this round, she said three rocks had fallen off. So I repeated the Setup with seven *remaining rocks*. Shortly, there was only one left. So I made the Setup:

I can keep this one rock, as I am so used to it.

On completing the round, however, there were no "rocks" left!

With regular tapping, Mrs. J. was gradually able to reduce pain and swelling. She reduced her medication to one painkiller a day and no sleeping pills. Her homeopath also started treatment. After about 2 weeks, he told her to consider dropping her painkiller and, if necessary, use paracetamol (in the U.S., acetaminophen, brand name Tylenol) instead.

She was highly troubled by this, as she felt she was dependent on the painkiller and, without it, the pain would be unbearable. We discussed the possible side effects of painkillers and I suggested we try tapping in the paracetamol as a substitute. She agreed.

So we did one round using:

Even though I think that only the prescription painkiller can provide relief from terrible pain, taking the paracetamol will prove to be equally effective for me.

Happily, she made the transition very smoothly and reported that the paracetamol worked as effectively as the strong painkiller she had been using. We plan to tap away her dependence on this pill after a couple of days. I think this may be a useful way to taper people off addictive and strong medications.

In our last session, after some discussion, she felt that she was facing an internal battle, where there was a part of her that wanted to return to complete health and another that felt attached to the disease, as it had served in getting attention from others and kept her family tied to her. (Fear of rejection is one of her major underlying emotional issues.)

I asked her to give this defiant part of herself a name and appearance. She called it "Inflexibility" and said it looked like a shadowy image of herself. We tapped for:

Even though Inflexibility does not want me to change and be well, I deeply and completely love, forgive, and accept myself.

She felt that the image was shrinking in size, until it looked like a small girl with two plaits, wearing a sari. Unsurprisingly, it reminded her of herself as a child. We next tapped on:

Even though Inflexibility has been staging this scary drama where I suffer a great deal of pain and I allowed myself to be conned by this play, I deeply and completely love, forgive, and accept myself.

This was followed by:

There is nothing to fear, I am safe and well.

In her mind, the little girl burst into tears, so I told her to hug her, and tapped:

Even though she scared me, she meant no harm. She was doing the best she knew. I deeply and completely love, forgive, and accept her.

At the end of this session, Mrs. J. was feeling substantially lighter, happier, and stronger. She felt optimistic about improvement and is now more motivated to fight her symptoms. Clearly, there is more work required, but there has certainly been noticeable improvement in her. I think the combination of EFT and homeopathy is proving to be highly effective for reducing her symptoms, in a relatively short time.

Update: I have been in regular touch with Mrs. J. over the past months. She is one of the most consistent and persistent tappers that I know. When I wrote the previous report 9 months ago, her rheumatoid factor was 72. She has been taking homeopathic treatment and continues with extensive tapping. In December 2007, seven months after she started tapping, her rheumatoid factor was down to 4. Her homeopathic doctor believes that she no longer has RA and her present symptoms are likely caused by cold weather and unresolved emotional issues.

Mrs. J. has unearthed many such emotional issues and has been working on various incidents and issues in her life. With the help of a pendulum and substance sensitivity charts, we found her to be sensitive to calcium and iron. After tapping for the same, she feels that her supplements are finally beginning to show a positive impact on her strength and energy. She has often noticed pain relief while tapping for issues related to forgiveness, rigidity, and resistance to change. On many occasions, Mrs. J. requires the Collarbone Breathing Exercise for Psychological Reversal.

Mrs. J. continues to have frequent episodes of stubborn pain and skin problems. Although there are many emotional and physical problems yet to be healed, she has already made incredible progress, and her commitment and faith in EFT is unshaken.

❋ ❋ ❋

Resources

Borrowing Benefits:
    BorrowingBenefits.EFTUniverse.com

Choices Method by Patricia Carrington:
    Choices.EFTUniverse.com

Collarbone Breathing:
    CollarboneBreathing.EFTUniverse.com

Core Issues and How to Find Them:
    CoreIssues.EFTUniverse.com

When Physical Symptoms Resist Healing:
    SymptomsResistHealing.EFTUniverse.com

12

Freedom from Pain
Through Forgiveness

We may intellectually understand that forgiveness is a good thing, but realizing that same fact emotionally can be a challenge. This may be so even after we give ourselves vivid demonstrations of how closely our pain is tied to anger, as was the case for Caroline, the school bus driver whose story you read in the last chapter. Some of us may even practice a religion that emphasizes forgiveness, yet we still endure the pain rather than let go of the anger.

If this is your situation, you may find it difficult if not impossible to tap through a Setup Statement that forgives the cause of your pain, such as:

Even though this pain gets worse when I think about my boss and how he treated me, I forgive him now.

Even though this pain gets worse whenever I think of how my sister betrayed me, I choose to forgive her and get on with my life.

*Even though it's hard to forgive him for what he did,
I know that holding on to my anger only makes the pain
worse, so I choose to forgive him now and let the pain go.*

*Even though I blame myself for this pain, I love and
forgive myself anyway.*

Forgiveness comes in many shades and, for some, forgiveness is impossible—at least for the time being. Some clients dig in their heels at the mere mention of "forgiving that bastard" and will go no further if forgiveness is the goal.

Add "Understanding"

Fortunately, the word "understand" carries less emotional baggage than the word "forgive," so adding it to the Setup Statement can help ease the transition from guilt or blame toward forgiveness and release.

*Even though this pain gets worse when I think about
my boss and how he treated me, I understand how this
all happened.*

*Even though this pain gets worse whenever I think
of how my sister betrayed me, I understand why she did
what she did.*

*Even though it's hard to forgive him for what he did,
I know that holding on to my anger only makes the pain
worse, so I choose to understand his situation now and
let the pain go.*

*Even though I blame myself for this pain, I understand why I did what I did, which was the best I could do
at the time.*

This substitution can help you switch mental gears and look at any situation differently. Whenever this happens while you are telling an old, familiar story, it's a clear indication that your emotional charge connected with the event is clearing. Any "cognitive shift," as psychologists call it, is a sign that EFT is working.

Release a Little Anger

Total forgiveness can seem like an impossible homework assignment. Fortunately, the simple strategy of giving up a little anger can go a long way toward releasing the rest. Some ways to do this are to project your release of anger far into the future or to make the whole project indefinite.

> *...I choose to know that I can some day release this anger.*

> *...I might someday, perhaps, forgive him a little.*

This all sounds very vague, but it replaces a flat "it's never going to happen" with the possibility of a future transformation.

Here is an important report from Dr. Patricia Carrington, who calls her elegant application of incremental EFT the "1% solution." This highly effective technique allows you to approach forgiveness by degrees.

Using EFT for Forgiveness:
The 1% Solution

by Patricia Carrington, PhD

I can't tell you how often people have told me that they simply cannot conceive of forgiving some other person for destructive acts that person has done—even if they use EFT for this problem. They feel that to do this would be paying mere lip service to the concept of "forgiveness." It would not come from their heart.

I agree that the act of "forgiveness" is all too often a pretense entered into by a person who feels obliged to "forgive" someone (or fate), perhaps for religious or ethical reasons. To truly forgive, especially when one feels resentment, fear, or anger about a "wrong" that has been done to self or others, is one of the most difficult and "unintuitive" things that we can do.

The reason for this may be the fact that the act of forgiving is not an act at all in any real sense. When it happens, it does so by default, as we let go of resentment against the other party along with the desire to punish.

Webster's New International Dictionary and the *Oxford Dictionary of the English Language* both define the verb "to forgive" as "to give up resentment against or the desire to punish; to stop being angry with; to pardon." It is quite clear that their definitions of forgiveness refer to the result of *letting go* of anger or resentment or desire for revenge. Forgiveness, then, is basically an *absence* of these negative emotions.

This makes for difficulty, however, when we attempt to use EFT to create forgiveness because it is much more difficult for people or animals to let go of something than it is for them to hold on to it. Ask someone, for example, to place a book on a table and, more than likely (if they have no particular reason for not doing so), they will find it easy to comply with your request, for they are being asked to do a direct and simple act.

Ask that same person to "let go" of a book they might already be holding, however, and they may well resist that request, or at least hesitate to carry it out until they give considerable thought to the consequences. They will probably consider possible outcomes that come to mind and will try to decide whether it is safe and advantageous for them to let go of the book. Perhaps it will fall on the floor and get damaged. Maybe the person will be "pushed around" or otherwise manipulated by you if they comply with this request. The result is that this person may be reluctant to let go of the book.

I am reminded of the way newborn infants show such a powerful grasp reflex. They can hold on with enormous strength to a finger or object within reach and not let go of it for a long time—sometimes their fingers have to be pried loose from the object. This grasp reflex may well be due to some inherited instinct that helped newborn humans to survive when we were tree-dwelling primates. It is likely that newborns had to be able to grasp onto their mothers or onto a tree branch to protect against a disastrous fall.

Whatever the reason, the fact is that it is usually easier for us to hold on to something than it is to let go of that same thing. Because of our use of language, we have a strong tendency to hold on to remembered wrongs and seemingly cannot pry ourselves loose from thoughts about "justice" and "punishment" for such wrongs. We cling to such thoughts tenaciously for long periods of time, sometimes for a lifetime. It is not surprising that we hear stories of vendettas that carry on from generation to generation in certain cultures, where a revenge motive actually controls the lives of the people caught in it.

How then can we bring about "forgiveness," which basically involves a *letting go* of resentment and giving up of the wish for revenge, even with the use of EFT?

Because forgiveness is actually something that happens automatically when resentment, anger, revenge, and a desire to punish have been relinquished, I am going to suggest a way in which EFT can be used to lessen or eliminate resentment and the punishment motive, thereby creating the natural state of forgiveness, which is, in fact, an absence of the need for revenge.

Since there is much reluctance in people to let go of resentment and the need for retribution, I have found it is far more productive to approach this matter in an indirect manner, little by little. One way I have found extremely effective is to break up the revenge motive into tiny manageable pieces. I call this the "Divide and Conquer" tactic. Here's how it works.

Suppose that Person A has been deeply hurt by Person B in the past. If you ask Person A to "forgive" Person B, it seems impossible at first. Even if you ask Person A to "let go" of any resentment he or she has toward Person B, it still tends to feel impossible. How, Person A reasons, can someone just let go of resentment if they've been deeply hurt?

A way to get around this trap, one which I find to be extraordinarily effective, is to break up the "letting go" process into tiny chunks, so you prove to yourself that your conviction that it's impossible to let go of your resentment isn't true, that resentment *can* be let go of in little pieces, which, of course, paves the way for a much greater letting go to come.

When you formulate your EFT statement, end the statement by a choice to "let go of only 1%" of your resentment. You can even add the phrase "and keep all the rest of it," if you wish. Here is how this statement might look in practice:

Even though I'm outraged at what he did, I choose to let go of 1% of my anger against him.

Even though I'm furious about what she did, I choose to release 1% of the rage I feel toward her.

If you use this "1% solution," you will probably have no trouble letting go of such a ridiculously small portion of your resentment. After all, it is not much to ask of yourself to give up 1% of it, and you are still allowed to retain most of your righteous anger!

However — and here is the secret in this approach — if you are able truly to let go of 1% of your resentment, anger, or desire to punish, then you will be in a very different state of mind than you were before. Something that seemed impossible will suddenly become possible, even if on a very small scale, and by letting it happen at all, you have actually opened a door to letting go of your resentments totally. A little release is always a big release. You will now have abandoned a deeply entrenched belief, a certainty that you *cannot* under any circumstances let go of your resentment!

I have many times seen this simple strategy result in a person's ability to entertain the *possibility* of letting go of *all* of their resentment. Once relinquishing a desire for revenge is seen as possible, the road has been cleared for you to release your entire resentment/punishment motive. When you let go of your tenacious hold on the conviction that "justice must be done at any cost," and punishment must be meted out for you to be at rest, you will finally be at rest. You will have lifted a tremendous emotional burden from yourself, and you'll be able to move ahead constructively with your life.

You may decide that you don't want to see that person again or put yourself in that kind of situation again, or you may decide to do so, according to rational decision. Either way, you are now free to choose what is really best for you. This is because the emotional charge has been removed from the situation. Now you will have "forgiven" that person in the true sense of that word. The revenge motive will have evaporated and, because unforgiveness depends on that motive, it too will have melted away. You will have forgiven this person or circumstance or fate in the true sense of the word, and can go on from there to build a new relationship, other better relationships, or whatever you desire.

I strongly recommend the "1% solution" when the need to forgive is resistant to any other approach.

❊ ❊ ❊

The EFT Gratitude Protocol

There is much to be grateful for, and when we adopt that state, many doors open. For example, filling the mind with gratitude leaves little room for unforgiveness, so if you're having trouble letting go of anger, blame, frustration, and other unforgiving emotions, try this approach. It's both easy and comfortable, and it can ease the transition toward complete forgiveness.

In tapping gratitude, you can use the whole Setup Statement, as in:

"Even though I'm angry at my boss for treating me that way last week, I am grateful for my job and all my boss has taught me,"

or go right to gratitude, tapping through the points while stating all that you are grateful for:

I'm grateful for my job, which allows me to make a living doing something I love.

I'm grateful that my boss recognizes my skills.

I'm grateful for my family and friends.

I'm grateful for all the love in my life.
I'm grateful for my musical talent.
I'm grateful for my health.

and so on.

Using EFT to tap on gratitude often produces unexpected shifts. You may find your anger and unwillingness to forgive evaporating as you tap. If it doesn't, you will likely feel better anyway. Tapping on gratitude tends to increase joy. Whatever your process, acknowledge any shift in how you feel by tapping your gratitude for that shift!

Angie Muccillo suggests applying gratitude to EFT itself. You can also modify her approach to use when you feel stuck or frustrated in your tapping, which may move you out of that state.

Tapping on Gratitude with EFT
by Angie Muccillo

Here's a simple little EFT protocol with the potential to increase EFT's effectiveness.

Are you grateful to EFT? I definitely am. I am grateful for not only the many positive effects it has had on my life personally, but also the many wondrous changes and healing I see in others as a result of using EFT. I think most people who have used EFT and achieved some degree of success with their personal and emotional issues have felt and expressed gratitude for what EFT has done for them. We have many documented accounts of these on the EFT website and in our clinics and offices worldwide.

EFT instructor Carol Tuttle recommends we tap on everything we are grateful for in our lives, as a way of focusing on what we have or want to attract more of. So, I thought, why not add EFT to that list? In essence, if we want to attract more success with our use of EFT, let's express our gratitude for it, like anything else. Carol also states, "Gratitude is one of the highest states of emotion we can experience." If we tap on our gratitude for EFT, we are focusing on our highest thoughts of EFT and placing our attention and thoughts on what we are grateful that EFT is doing for us. In other words, we use the EFT affirmation to affirm EFT!

The idea is simply to use the EFT Gratitude Protocol at the end (or beginning) of a tapping session with a round or two of statements focused on your gratitude toward EFT. I think giving thanks to EFT is a kind of pleasant and harmonious way to open or close a tapping session, whether it is with a practitioner or on your own.

Whether the session has completely resolved your issues or not, inserting the Gratitude Protocol at the end may set a positive scene for future tapping and perhaps help build a bridge to the next session. I would also recommend using the Gratitude Protocol routinely as a daily or homework exercise or when you feel stuck.

EFT Gratitude Statements

Tap the EFT points while repeating each statement:

I am deeply and completely grateful for EFT.

I am deeply and completely grateful for releasing these emotions with EFT.

I am deeply and completely grateful for the ease with which EFT is helping me to release my fears, phobias, and traumatic memories.

I am deeply and completely grateful to EFT for relieving my back/shoulder pain.

I am deeply and completely grateful for the ease with which EFT is helping me to release my addictions.

I am deeply and completely grateful that I have EFT to help me release my pain and suffering.

I am deeply and completely grateful for the ease with which EFT works for me each and every time.

I am deeply and completely grateful that I have a tool to help me calm down whenever I need it.

I am deeply and completely grateful for the positive changes EFT has helped me make in my life.

I am deeply and completely grateful for the many benefits I am receiving from using EFT daily.

I am deeply and completely grateful for the positive impact EFT is having on my life and those around me.

I am deeply and completely grateful for the peace and calm EFT has brought into my life.

I am deeply and completely grateful to EFT for improving the quality of my life.

I am deeply and completely grateful I have discovered this wonderful tool!

These are just a few suggestions. I am sure there's a lot of gratitude out there for EFT! Let's hear it and share it. As a general rule, write your statements as though your EFT goals have already been achieved.

This protocol can also be useful when EFT "doesn't appear to be working" or you feel stuck or frustrated. Although there are many one-minute wonders in EFT, as we know, some issues take time to break down and, in the process, you can find yourself getting frustrated, overwhelmed, even unappreciative and forgetful of the progress you have actually made. You can use this protocol to help break free from some of these barriers by switching your thinking to what you are grateful for instead. You can use the Choices Method to install gratitude.

Sample Setups

Even though EFT isn't working for my back pain yet, I choose to be grateful to EFT for helping me release these emotions and for all the healing I have achieved so far.

Even though I don't get the same results as Mary did, I choose to be grateful I have a tool to help me calm down whenever I need it.

Even though I'm sick of tapping and don't seem to be getting anywhere, I am grateful for the positive changes EFT has helped me make in my life.

What are you grateful for when it comes to EFT? Write your list of gratitude statements and tap on them regularly.

❀ ❀ ❀

Resources

Choices Method by Patricia Carrington: Choices.EFTUniverse.com

Practitioners: Practitioners.EFTUniverse.com

Relationship Stories: RelationshipStories.EFTUniverse.com

Spirituality Stories: SpiritualityStories.EFTUniverse.com

Submit Your EFT Story to Archives: SubmitStory.EFTuniverse.com

Tapping Circles: TappingCircles.EFTUniverse.com

Work Stories: WorkStories.EFTUniverse.com

In Conclusion

Thank you for trusting me as your guide through the process of finding solutions to your back pain. I hope that you are experiencing a lot less pain now than when you first began reading this book. I know that though I have to be conscious of my movement every day, I'm no longer periodically crippled by back pain the way I was before discovering the methods we've been reviewing in these pages. What you have experienced is just the start. There are many more benefits to EFT that will emerge as you maintain a consistent practice. It is easy to forget about EFT after you get relief, so I encourage you to make it part of your daily routine. Tap when you wake up and review your intentions for the day. Tap before you go to bed as you visualize a good night's sleep. Tap any time in between when you are emotionally triggered, so you give yourself a baseline state of emotional peace.

Use the many resources EFT has to offer. Take our online EFT for First Aid course at TraumaTap.com. Find a practitioner to work with, especially on those issues that seem too difficult to work on alone. If you need help losing weight, use the many resources at WeightLoss. EFTuniverse.com. Take one of our weekend workshops. From an expert certified trainer, you will learn the fundamentals of EFT from the ground up, and make great personal connections while doing so. Read the stories published at EFTuniverse.com, and write and tell us your own success stories. Above all, never accept that your life has to be limited. I sincerely want to see you live an abundant, healthy, and happy life. Thanks for joining me on this journey. I look forward to seeing you at the next stage of wellness!

References

Adams, A., & Davidson, K. (2011). *EFT comprehensive training resource level 1.* Santa Rosa, CA: Energy Psychology Press.

Borenstein, D. G., O'Mara, J. W., Jr., Boden, S. D., Lauerman, W. C., Jacobson, A., Platenberg, C., Schellinger, D., & Wiesel, S. W. (2001, September). The value of magnetic resonance imaging of the lumbar spine to predict low-back pain in asymptomatic subjects: A seven-year follow-up study. *Journal of Bone and Joint Surgery, 83-A*(9), 1306–1311.

Bougea, A. M., Spandideas, N., Alexopoulos, E. C., Thomaides, T., Chrousos, G. P., & Darviri, C. (2013). Effect of the Emotional Freedom Technique on perceived stress, quality of life, and cortisol salivary levels in tension-type headache sufferers: A randomized controlled trial. *Explore: The Journal of Science and Healing, 9*(2), 91–99. doi:10.1016/j.explore.2012.12.005.

Brody, J. (2007). Living with pain that just won't go away. *New York Times,* November 6, 2007.

Callahan, R. (2000). *Tapping the healer within: Using Thought Field Therapy to instantly conquer your fears, anxieties, and emotional distress.* New York, NY: McGraw-Hill.

Chambless, D., Baker, M. J., Baucom, D. H., Beutler, L. E., Calhoun, K. S., Crits-Christoph, P.,… Woody, S. R. (1998). Update on empirically validated therapies, II. *Clinical Psychologist, 51,* 3–16.

Chambless, D., & Hollon, S. D. (1998). Defining empirically supported therapies. *Journal of Consulting and Clinical Psychology, 66,* 7–18.

Chambless, D. L., Sanderson, W. C., Shoham, V., Bennett Johnson, S., Pope, K. S., Crits-Christoph, P.,… McCurry, C. (1996). An update on empirically validated therapies. *Clinical Psychologist, 49,* 5–18.

Cherkin, D. C., Sherman, K. J., Avins, A. L., Erro, J. H., Ichikawa, L., Barlow, W. E.,… Deyo, R. A. (2009, May 11). A randomized trial comparing acupuncture, simulated acupuncture, and usual care for chronic low back pain. *Archives of Internal Medicine, 169*(9), 858–866. doi:10.1001/archinternmed.2009.65

Church, D. (2013). *The EFT manual* (3rd ed.). Santa Rosa, CA: Energy Psychology Press.

Church, D. (2014). Pain, depression, and anxiety after PTSD symptom remediation in veterans. *Explore: The Journal of Science and Healing* (in press).

Church, D., & Brooks, A. J. (2010). The effect of a brief EFT (Emotional Freedom Techniques) self-intervention on anxiety, depression, pain and cravings in healthcare workers. *Integrative Medicine: A Clinician's Journal, 9*(4), 40–44.

Church, D., Hawk, C., Brooks, A., Toukolehto, O., Wren, M., Dinter, I., & Stein, P. (2013). Psycho-logical trauma symptom improvement in veterans using EFT (Emotional Freedom Techniques): A randomized controlled trial. *Journal of Nervous and Mental Disease, 201,* 153–160.

Craig, G., & Fowlie, A. (1995). *Emotional freedom techniques: The manual.* Sea Ranch, CA: Gary Craig.

Diepold, J. H., & Goldstein, D. (2008). Thought Field Therapy and qEEG changes in the treatment of trauma: A case study. *Traumatology, 15*(1), 85–93. http://dx.doi.org/10.1177/1534765608325304

Eden, D. (with Feinstein, D.). (2008). *Energy medicine: Balancing your body's energies for optimal health, joy, and vitality* (2nd ed.). New York, NY: Tarcher/Penguin.

Feinstein, D. (2012). Acupoint stimulation in treating psychological disorders: Evidence of efficacy. *Review of General Psychology, 16*(4), 364–380. doi:10.1037/a0028602

Feinstein, D., Eden, D., & Craig, G. (2005). *The promise of energy psychology: Revolutionary tools for dramatic personal change.* New York, NY: Jeremy P. Tarcher/Penguin.

Grant, M. (2009). *Change your brain, change your pain.* Wyong, NSW, Australia: Mark Grant.

Katie, B. (2002). *Loving what is: Four questions that can change your life.* New York, NY: Harmony Books.

Lambrou, P. T., Pratt, G. J., & Chevalier, G. (2003). Physiological and psychological effects of a mind/body therapy on claustrophobia. *Subtle Energies and Energy Medicine, 14,* 239–251.

Phelps, E. A., & LeDoux, J. E. (2005). Contributions of the amygdala to emotion processing: From animal models to human behavior. *Neuron, 48,* 175–187.

Rogers, C. R. (1961). *On becoming a person: A therapist's view of psychotherapy.* New York, NY: Houghton Mifflin.

Sarno, J. E. (2006). *The divided mind: The epidemic of mindbody disorders.* New York, NY: Regan Books.

Schneider, J. (2009). *Living with chronic pain: The complete health guide to the causes and treatment of chronic pain* (2nd ed.). Long Island City, NY: Hatherleigh Press.

Swingle, P. G., Pulos, L., & Swingle, M. K. (2004). Neuro-physiological indicators of EFT treatment of posttraumatic stress. *Subtle Energies and Energy Medicine, 15*(1), 75–86.

Vickers, A. J., Cronin, A. M., Maschino, A. C., Lewith, G., MacPherson, H., Foster, N. E.,… Linde, K. (2012, October 22). Acupuncture for chronic pain: Individual patient data meta-analysis. *Archives of Internal Medicine, 172*(19), 1444–1453. doi:10.1001/archinternmed.2012.3654

Wolpe, J. (1958). *Psychotherapy by reciprocal inhibition.* Palo Alto, CA: Stanford University Press.

EFT Resources

For information about EFT, including a free down-loadable Get Started package, go to www.EFTUniverse.com. On this website, you'll find thousands of case histories of people who've used EFT successfully for every conceivable problem. You'll also find practitioner listings, tutorials, books, DVDs, classes, volunteer opportunities, and other resources to allow you to get the most from EFT.

Index